New Mama
Celebration Planner

New Mama Celebration Planner
Copyright © 2022 by Thrive Femme Designs

All rights reserved. No part of this publication may be reproduced, distributed, or transmitted in any form or by any means, including photocopying, recording, or other electronic or mechanical methods, without the prior written permission of the author, except in the case of brief quotations embodied in critical reviews and certain other non-commercial uses permitted by copyright law.

The author and publisher make no representation or warranties with respect to the accuracy, applicability, or completeness of the contents herein. The information and strategies contained herein may not be suitable for your situation. Neither the author, nor the publisher shall be liable for damages arising from this book or its contents. Therefore, if you wish to apply the ideas contained herein, you take full responsibility for your actions. Always seek the advice of a physician or other qualified health provider properly licensed to practice medicine or general health care concerning any questions you may have regarding any information obtained herein. The use of this book implies your acceptance of this disclaimer.

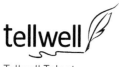

Tellwell Talent
www.tellwell.ca

ISBN
978-0-2288-7600-7 (Hardcover)
978-0-2288-7599-4 (Paperback)

New Mama Name:

_____

Mama Born On:

_____

Baby's Name:

_____

Table of Contents

Welcome, Mama!..1

    Let's celebrate YOU!...1

    Our Story..3

    Getting the most from your New Mama Celebration Planner!......5

Part I   Preparation for motherhood..9

    Beginning Your Journey..10

    Setting Intentions for Postpartum..11

    Postpartum Resources...12

    JOY-FULL List: Things that Light You Up!.......................................14

Part II   Welcome to motherhood...17

    Welcome, mama!..18

    Affirmations..19

Part III   New Mama Celebration Planner......................................21

    Monthly Wellbeing Check-in

    Monthly Calendar

    What's happening this week

    Daily planner pages

    Monthly Recap

Let's Celebrate!..191

Welcome, Mama!

Let's celebrate YOU!

Congratulations! I am thrilled you have your *New Mama Celebration Planner* in your hands! It was created with love to support you to THRIVE through your postpartum journey.

The journey of a human becoming a human who is also a mama is a unique experience for each and every person. Your experience is valid. It is your own. It is part of your story, and it is happening *for* you.

Motherhood can feel like a rollercoaster, and we want you to know you're not alone on the ride. Although there may be times when it doesn't feel like it, know that you are seen for the magnificent human you are. Even when it may feel as though you're only giving love, know that you are loved beyond measure. You are worthy of being celebrated each and every day: in the small, mundane moments, when the grand milestones are reached, and everywhere in between.

Together, we THRIVE!

Our Story

The New Mama Celebration Planner came to form as I reconnected with my inner purpose after becoming a mother. This is the purpose that lights me up and gets me excited to get out of bed in the morning, the one I had prior to becoming a human who is also a mama. I say it this way because after my first child, I felt as though I lost myself in motherhood. Everything was about my baby, everything felt as though I was supposed to be fulfilling my duties and other roles in life. I put myself at the bottom of the care list. My basic needs were met, and not much else. After experiencing postpartum anxiety, I recognized my anxious feelings stemmed from a belief I held (a belief many of us have from society as we enter motherhood) that I was supposed to be able to do everything alone. I started reaching out for support. I turned within and started to ask myself "What do I need?"

I started journaling about these inner truths. I wrote about what I was feeling and what I thought could help and started sharing that with those who could support me. I will note that reaching out for help did not come easily to me. I had spent the majority of my life priding myself on the notion of being strong and independent. Releasing myself of that narrative and receiving support made the greatest impact on my mental health and I desire this for you too.

This planner has been created with the intention to help you connect with YOU, to guide and support you as you honour yourself and your needs so you can THRIVE. By following the prompts throughout this planner, it is my hope that you will get to know yourself on a deeper level. You will bring into your awareness things that bring you joy, things you're grateful for, ways you like to be supported, how you speak to yourself, etc. It is the goal of this planner for you to celebrate you and your inner truth as you navigate your unique journey into motherhood and beyond.

I see you. I love you. I hold space for you. I celebrate you!

With Love & Gratitude,

Heather xo

We love to celebrate you!
Tag us @nakedtank to be featured through your New Mama journey.

Getting the most from your New Mama Celebration Planner!

This is your celebration planner! It is here to support and guide you to celebrate yourself as you prepare for postpartum and navigate your first year (and beyond) in motherhood.

PART I: Preparation for motherhood

You've probably spent a great amount of time during pregnancy preparing for the birth of your baby. Yes, the crib may be set up and the clothes may be washed and ready for your little one's arrival, but what about you? In this section, we encourage you to take some quiet time before your baby's arrival to write out your feelings. Make a plan on paper for what you desire postpartum to look and feel like for you.

Review and fill in the resource prompts to set yourself up with support contacts so you have them on hand as needed. Have fun writing your JOY-FULL list with activities that light you up for quick reference on a postpartum day. Wrap yourself in comfort and peace with these steps as you prepare yourself, mind, body, and soul, for postpartum.

PART II: Welcome to motherhood

Here, we welcome you to motherhood. We invite you to write your birth story and affirm yourself as the glorious human and mother that you are.

PART III: New Mama Celebration Planner

Monthly: Bring ease and order to your postpartum mind. Record upcoming special dates, events, appointments, and milestones in your monthly calendar. On your monthly wellbeing check-in, connect with yourself and make a plan to support how you desire to feel each month. Recap your growth and celebrate at the end of each month.

Weekly: Set yourself up for the week with your "What's happening this week?" planner page. Set reminders for events to celebrate that are coming up this week and write out grocery items as they come to you in the space provided so you can snap a picture before the next shopping trip.

Daily Celebration and Reflection: Show yourself some LOVE each morning! Start your day with a pep talk, gratitude, and a quick plan for your daily wellbeing. Finish the day with reflection and celebration.

Affirmations: Each week (or day if you prefer), write an affirmation at the top of your daily planner page. Write something that feels good to you. Make it your own; you are affirming who you are with these simple statements. Think of them as gentle reminders that help keep your head and heart steady throughout the day. All that you need already lies within you.

Habit Tracker: Track a habit that you desire to integrate into your life. Keep it simple. This is a reminder to focus on something for YOU each day and make that a habit. You can't pour from an empty cup, so it's important to honour yourself. No habit is too small. (HINT: a great kickstart habit: fill in the daily planner for thirty days.)

Sample Daily Planner Page

Morning PEP TALK

- ∞ In the mirror, with one hand on your heart: I LOVE YOU. YOU'VE GOT THIS, _____ Heather _____!
  (NAME)
- ∞ Affirmation: I (AM) _The best mother for my baby_
- ∞ I am grateful for (3+) _The sleep/rest I did get last night, my connection with my baby getting stronger, the sunshine_
- ∞ I thank my body for _Supporting me as I heal._
- ∞ HABIT TRACKER, Day _1_ of 30

Wellbeing ACTIONS

- ☑ Today, I GET to _Play my favourite song_ for me (prompts: JOY-FULL List p.15)
- ☐ Today, I GET to _Snuggle with_ my baby.
- ☑ Today, I GET to _Share my win_ for/with _My partner_
  (e.g., spouse, kids, friends)

Nighttime REFLECTION

- ∞ WIN: I am _Celebrating_ myself for _Taking a nap while the baby napped_
- ∞ CHALLENGE: It felt hard when _My baby cried_
  - ♥ I choose to see this as an opportunity to _Learn about my baby_
  - ♥ Say aloud: *I forgive, and I release this challenge with love. *Inhale, Exhale**
- ∞ SUPPORT: I felt supported today by/when _I had energy boosting snacks on hand_
- ∞ GRATITUDE: I am grateful for _My body healing, feeding my baby, roof over our head_
- ∞ INTENTION: My intention for the morning is _Take things slow_

Part 1
Preparation for motherhood

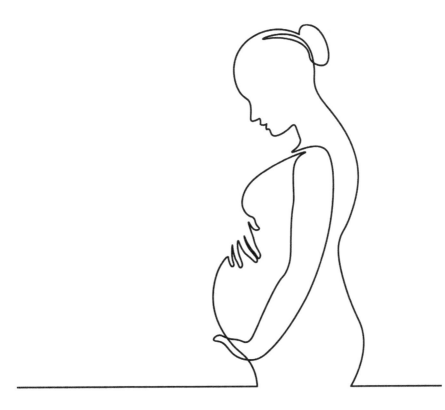

Beginning Your Journey

How are you feeling? Know that you are not alone in this journey. Honour your feelings and take comfort in knowing that around the world, there are mamas experiencing the same joys and fears in their lives as they navigate this journey alongside you.

There is no such thing as perfect in parenthood. I invite you to give yourself permission to release even attempting perfection. Find peace in knowing that you have everything you need within you to be the best parent for your child. You are enough as you are, and you get to learn new things along the way.

Loving your child starts within. We set the example for our little ones, and it is an incredible gift to influence a child intimately as your adventures of life continue. Show yourself grace. Trust you are doing your best with what you have, and your best is enough. To love others with our whole heart, we get to love ourselves with our whole heart as well.

Begin this journey with three little words you say to the most important person in your world – YOU! These three words are: I LOVE YOU. Pause, close your eyes, put your hands on your chest, inhale, exhale, and say it out loud to yourself: "I LOVE YOU." Feel that feeling being true throughout your whole body.

Free write:

_____

_____

_____

_____

You've got this, Mama!

Setting Intentions for Postpartum

Ask yourself:

1. How do I desire to feel in my first year postpartum? (Prompts: energy, sleep, nourishment, movement, hygiene, body image, connection with baby, etc.)

_____

_____

_____

_____

2. What action steps can I take NOW to prepare to feel supported in these areas during postpartum?

   ACTION 1: _____

   ACTION 2: _____

   ACTION 3: _____

   ACTION 4: _____

3. When did I feel accomplished? What experience did I feel I was getting the results I wanted? Go back to that time, imagine I'm living it again in this moment. Describe this situation in as much detail as possible, including the feelings I felt. **Note: Flag this page for reference when you're feeling low. Connect the feelings from this accomplished experience into the present moment.**

I felt accomplished when _____

_____

_____

_____

Postpartum Resources

Let's prepare you with accessible resources to support you and your baby throughout your postpartum journey. Feel safe with contacts that you can reach out to for help. *You are not alone!*

<u>Please do not skip this section!</u> Surround yourself with support! Knowing the resources available to you postpartum can give you peace of mind before your baby's arrival. This can help you respond to your postpartum experiences with more ease.

Many mamas before you have felt motherhood to, paradoxically, feel like the loneliest time in the world even though they're very close with another person (baby) for the majority of their days. Our mission with *The New Mama Celebration Planner* is to support YOU with tools to help you THRIVE as a human, a woman, a mother, and more. *You are worthy as you are!*

Celebrate being open and prepared to receive support and care during this time!

Use this space to record the contact information of a trusted loved one and health professionals who are available to help in your region either in-person or virtually.

Resources:	Name	Contact Information
Trusted Loved One:	_____	_____
OB/Midwife:	_____	_____
Postpartum Doula:	_____	_____
Licensed Lactation Consultant:	_____	_____
Pelvic Health Physiotherapist:	_____	_____
Psychologist/Counsellor:	_____	_____

Registered Massage Therapist* _____   _____

Family Physician: _____   _____

Other: _____ _____   _____

Other: _____ _____   _____

*pre/postnatal certified recommended

JOY-FULL List:
Things that Light You Up!

I see you, Mama. Society tends to focus on Mama being comfy and well during pregnancy, and then all eyes are on the baby once your baby arrives. Yes, your baby is relying on you to meet the majority of their needs throughout the days and nights, and that is an important role to fulfil, and that doesn't mean you should drop yourself to the bottom of the care list. Remember, YOU have been born into this new role, this body transformed – your needs and desires are valid and important. When you feel good from the inside-out, you show up differently, and this can enhance your connection to your baby (and those around you).

We each have a vibrational frequency that our emotions/energy may resonate with. You have a power within you to shift your vibration at any moment you choose. When you have things top of mind that support you feeling high vibration emotions, such as joy, love, gratitude, empowerment, etc., you can experience a positive shift in your energy, and your baby's behaviour may reflect that.

<u>Exercise</u>: Take a few moments to think about a time you felt pure JOY in your life. Inhale, exhale, see the experience playing in your mind, getting your senses involved. Hold that feeling.

What came to mind? What activities or thoughts bring you good feelings from the inside-out? Include things that you can do anywhere with your body alone, such as deep breaths, a shower/bath, your favourite music, going for a walk. **Note: Flag this page for easy reference during your daily planner to prompt ideas for what you get to do for YOU each day.**

Disclaimer: See your healthcare practitioner before beginning physical activity and/or if you are unsure about engaging in a certain activity postpartum.

Notes

Part II
Welcome to motherhood

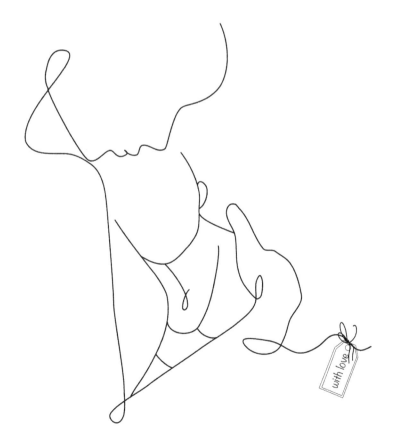

Welcome, mama!

As a twist on the classic baby books that share the birth story of your little one and give space to record and celebrate their milestones, *The New Mama Celebration Planner* invites you to write your personal rebirth story as you transform into a human who is also a mother. You define that moment/journey for you.

This is your story; it is unique to you. There is no right or wrong. Write from your heart and celebrate yourself.

My Birth Story:

_____

_____

_____

_____

_____

_____

_____

_____

_____

_____

_____

_____

_____

_____

Affirmations

The New Mama Celebration Planner is here to bring ease, joy, and confidence to your postpartum experience. Repeating affirmations to yourself while holding the feeling of them can give you an emotional boost to support you through your days and weeks. Trust that you are right where you're supposed to be. You are enough. **Note: Reach out to your Resources list on p.12-13 if you feel something isn't right.** It takes courage to reach out for help; we are not meant to take on motherhood alone.

You can use the positive statements below or create your own. Believe that they are already your truth. Write, read, and/or say them often to let these truths shine through. The power is in the feeling behind the words. TIP: Write them on post-it notes and put them around your home.

- ♥ I AM DEEPLY SUPPORTED. I ACCEPT THE HELP OF OTHERS.
- ♥ I AM THE BEST MOTHER FOR MY BABY.
- ♥ I TRUST MY INSTINCTS TO KNOW WHAT'S BEST FOR MY BABY.
- ♥ I AM CONNECTING TO MY BABY MORE DEEPLY EVERY DAY.
- ♥ I GIVE MYSELF GRACE, TODAY, AND EVERY DAY.
- ♥ I AM PATIENT WITH MYSELF AND MY BABY.
- ♥ I HONOUR MY BODY FOR ALL IT HAS DONE AND IS DOING FOR ME.
- ♥ I AM ENOUGH; WHAT I DO IS ENOUGH.
- ♥ I AM LOVE. I GIVE LOVE, AND I RECEIVE LOVE.
- ♥ I _____
- ♥ I _____
- ♥ I _____

Notes

Part III
New Mama Celebration Planner

MONTH: _____

SUNDAY	MONDAY	TUESDAY	WEDNESDAY
___	___	___	___
___	___	___	___
___	___	___	___
___	___	___	___
___	___	___	___

Record special dates, appointments, milestones, etc.

THURSDAY	FRIDAY	SATURDAY	NOTES
___	___	___	
___	___	___	
___	___	___	
___	___	___	
___	___	___	

Monthly Wellbeing Check-in

MONTH: _____

1. How do I feel right now?
    - ◊ In my head (mentally): _____
    _____
    - ◊ In my heart (emotionally): _____
    _____
    - ◊ In my body (physically): _____
    _____

2. How do I desire to feel?
    - ◊ In my head (mentally): _____
    _____
    - ◊ In my heart (emotionally): _____
    _____
    - ◊ In my body (physically): _____
    _____

3. What actions can I take to help me feel the way I described above? What thoughts can I have to help me feel this way?
    - ◊ In my head (mentally): _____
    _____
    - ◊ In my heart (emotionally): _____
    _____
    - ◊ In my body (physically): _____
    _____

4. What am I excited for this month? _____

_____

5. What boundary am I setting up this month? _____

_____

   ◊   Action(s) to set up this boundary: _____

       _____

6. HABIT TRACKER (e.g., action/thought you wrote about for your desired feeling in #3):

I _____ am developing the habit of _____ this month.
  (NAME)

Picture this as a habit already. How do I feel? How am I showing up? What is different?

_____

_____

_____

_____

_____

_____

I understand that I may miss a day. I will show myself grace and re-commit the next day.

This habit supports me.

I am doing my best and I am Thriving!

What's happening this week

Week of: _____

- ♥ Affirmation: I _____

- ♥ I will show myself grace this week by _____

- ♥ I am looking forward to _____

- ♥ I get to ask for support with _____

    By (action step) _____

- ☐ Review #2-6 from the Monthly Wellbeing Check-in. Take a moment to visualize yourself integrating these feelings, actions, and thoughts now, as well as throughout this week.

- ☐ Review upcoming appointments and set an alarm in your phone as needed.

Grocery list:
(TIP: Record here and take a picture to bring ease to the next grocery store trip.)

_____	_____	_____
_____	_____	_____
_____	_____	_____
_____	_____	_____
_____	_____	_____
_____	_____	_____
_____	_____	_____

Monday

Morning PEP TALK

- ∞ In the mirror, with one hand on your heart: I LOVE YOU. YOU'VE GOT THIS, _____ !
  (NAME)
- ∞ Affirmation: I (AM) _____
- ∞ I am grateful for (3+) _____
  _____
- ∞ I thank my body for _____
- ∞ HABIT TRACKER, Day ___ of 30

Wellbeing ACTIONS

- ☐ Today, I GET to _____ for me (prompts: JOY-FULL List p.15)
- ☐ Today, I GET to _____ my baby.
- ☐ Today, I GET to _____ for/with _____
  (e.g., spouse, kids, friends)

Nighttime REFLECTION

- ∞ WIN: I am *Celebrating* myself for _____
- ∞ CHALLENGE: It felt hard when _____
  - ♥ I choose to see this as an opportunity to _____
  - ♥ Say aloud: *I forgive, and I release this challenge with love. *Inhale, Exhale**
- ∞ SUPPORT: I felt supported today by/when _____
  _____
- ∞ GRATITUDE: I am grateful for _____
  _____
- ∞ INTENTION: My intention for the morning is _____

Tuesday

Morning PEP TALK

- ∞ In the mirror, with one hand on your heart: I LOVE YOU. YOU'VE GOT THIS, _____!
  (NAME)
- ∞ Affirmation: I (AM) _____
- ∞ I am grateful for (3+) _____
  _____
- ∞ I thank my body for _____
- ∞ HABIT TRACKER, Day ___ of 30

Wellbeing ACTIONS

- ☐ Today, I GET to _____ for me (prompts: JOY-FULL List p.15)
- ☐ Today, I GET to _____ my baby.
- ☐ Today, I GET to _____ for/with _____
  (e.g., spouse, kids, friends)

Nighttime REFLECTION

- ∞ WIN: I am _Celebrating_ myself for _____
- ∞ CHALLENGE: It felt hard when _____
  - ♥ I choose to see this as an opportunity to _____
  - ♥ Say aloud: *I forgive, and I release this challenge with love. *Inhale, Exhale**
- ∞ SUPPORT: I felt supported today by/when _____
  _____
- ∞ GRATITUDE: I am grateful for _____
  _____
- ∞ INTENTION: My intention for the morning is _____

Wednesday

Morning PEP TALK

- ∞ In the mirror, with one hand on your heart: I LOVE YOU. YOU'VE GOT THIS, _____!
  (NAME)
- ∞ Affirmation: I (AM) _____
- ∞ I am grateful for (3+) _____
  _____
- ∞ I thank my body for _____
- ∞ HABIT TRACKER, Day ___ of 30

Wellbeing ACTIONS

- ☐ Today, I GET to _____ for me (prompts: JOY-FULL List p.15)
- ☐ Today, I GET to _____ my baby.
- ☐ Today, I GET to _____ for/with _____
  (e.g., spouse, kids, friends)

Nighttime REFLECTION

- ∞ WIN: I am *Celebrating* myself for _____
- ∞ CHALLENGE: It felt hard when _____
  - ♥ I choose to see this as an opportunity to _____
  - ♥ Say aloud: *I forgive, and I release this challenge with love. *Inhale, Exhale**
- ∞ SUPPORT: I felt supported today by/when _____
  _____
- ∞ GRATITUDE: I am grateful for _____
  _____
- ∞ INTENTION: My intention for the morning is _____

Thursday

Morning PEP TALK

- ∞ In the mirror, with one hand on your heart: I LOVE YOU. YOU'VE GOT THIS, _____!
  (NAME)
- ∞ Affirmation: I (AM) _____
- ∞ I am grateful for (3+) _____
  _____
- ∞ I thank my body for _____
- ∞ HABIT TRACKER, Day ___ of 30

Wellbeing ACTIONS

- ☐ Today, I GET to _____ for me (prompts: JOY-FULL List p.15)
- ☐ Today, I GET to _____ my baby.
- ☐ Today, I GET to _____ for/with _____
  (e.g., spouse, kids, friends)

Nighttime REFLECTION

- ∞ WIN: I am _Celebrating_ myself for _____
- ∞ CHALLENGE: It felt hard when _____
  - ♥ I choose to see this as an opportunity to _____
  - ♥ Say aloud: *I forgive, and I release this challenge with love.* *Inhale, Exhale*
- ∞ SUPPORT: I felt supported today by/when _____
  _____
- ∞ GRATITUDE: I am grateful for _____
  _____
- ∞ INTENTION: My intention for the morning is _____

Friday

Morning PEP TALK

- ∞ In the mirror, with one hand on your heart: I LOVE YOU. YOU'VE GOT THIS, _____!
  (NAME)
- ∞ Affirmation: I (AM) _____
- ∞ I am grateful for (3+) _____
  _____
- ∞ I thank my body for _____
- ∞ HABIT TRACKER, Day ___ of 30

Wellbeing ACTIONS

- ☐ Today, I GET to _____ for me (prompts: JOY-FULL List p.15)
- ☐ Today, I GET to _____ my baby.
- ☐ Today, I GET to _____ for/with _____
  (e.g., spouse, kids, friends)

Nighttime REFLECTION

- ∞ WIN: I am *Celebrating* myself for _____
- ∞ CHALLENGE: It felt hard when _____
  - ♥ I choose to see this as an opportunity to _____
  - ♥ Say aloud: *I forgive, and I release this challenge with love. *Inhale, Exhale**
- ∞ SUPPORT: I felt supported today by/when _____
  _____
- ∞ GRATITUDE: I am grateful for _____
  _____
- ∞ INTENTION: My intention for the morning is _____

Saturday

Morning PEP TALK

- ∞ In the mirror, with one hand on your heart: I LOVE YOU. YOU'VE GOT THIS, _____!
  (NAME)
- ∞ Affirmation: I (AM) _____
- ∞ I am grateful for (3+) _____
  _____
- ∞ I thank my body for _____
- ∞ HABIT TRACKER, Day ___ of 30

Wellbeing ACTIONS

- ☐ Today, I GET to _____ for me (prompts: JOY-FULL List p.15)
- ☐ Today, I GET to _____ my baby.
- ☐ Today, I GET to _____ for/with _____
  (e.g., spouse, kids, friends)

Nighttime REFLECTION

- ∞ WIN: I am *Celebrating* myself for _____
- ∞ CHALLENGE: It felt hard when _____
  - ♥ I choose to see this as an opportunity to _____
  - ♥ Say aloud: *I forgive, and I release this challenge with love. *Inhale, Exhale**
- ∞ SUPPORT: I felt supported today by/when _____
  _____
- ∞ GRATITUDE: I am grateful for _____
  _____
- ∞ INTENTION: My intention for the morning is _____

Sunday

Morning PEP TALK

- ∞ In the mirror, with one hand on your heart: I LOVE YOU. YOU'VE GOT THIS, _____!
  _(NAME)
- ∞ Affirmation: I (AM) _____
- ∞ I am grateful for (3+) _____
- ∞ I thank my body for _____
- ∞ HABIT TRACKER, Day ___ of 30

Wellbeing ACTIONS

- ☐ Today, I GET to _____ for me (prompts: JOY-FULL List p.15)
- ☐ Today, I GET to _____ my baby.
- ☐ Today, I GET to _____ for/with _____
  _(e.g., spouse, kids, friends)

Nighttime REFLECTION

- ∞ WIN: I am *Celebrating* myself for _____
- ∞ CHALLENGE: It felt hard when _____
  - ♥ I choose to see this as an opportunity to _____
  - ♥ Say aloud: *I forgive, and I release this challenge with love. *Inhale, Exhale**
- ∞ SUPPORT: I felt supported today by/when _____
- ∞ GRATITUDE: I am grateful for _____
- ∞ INTENTION: My intention for the morning is _____

What's happening this week

Week of: _____

- ♥ Affirmation: I _____

- ♥ I will show myself grace this week by _____

- ♥ I am looking forward to _____

- ♥ I get to ask for support with _____

    By (action step) _____

- ☐ Review #2-6 from the Monthly Wellbeing Check-in. Take a moment to visualize yourself integrating these feelings, actions, and thoughts now, as well as throughout this week.

- ☐ Review upcoming appointments and set an alarm in your phone as needed.

Grocery list:
(TIP: Record here and take a picture to bring ease to the next grocery store trip.)

_____	_____	_____
_____	_____	_____
_____	_____	_____
_____	_____	_____
_____	_____	_____
_____	_____	_____
_____	_____	_____

Monday

Morning PEP TALK

- ∞ In the mirror, with one hand on your heart: I LOVE YOU. YOU'VE GOT THIS, _____ !
  (NAME)
- ∞ Affirmation: I (AM) _____
- ∞ I am grateful for (3+) _____
  _____
- ∞ I thank my body for _____
- ∞ HABIT TRACKER, Day ___ of 30

Wellbeing ACTIONS

- ☐ Today, I GET to _____ for me (prompts: JOY-FULL List p.15)
- ☐ Today, I GET to _____ my baby.
- ☐ Today, I GET to _____ for/with _____
  (e.g., spouse, kids, friends)

Nighttime REFLECTION

- ∞ WIN: I am *Celebrating* myself for _____
- ∞ CHALLENGE: It felt hard when _____
  - ♥ I choose to see this as an opportunity to _____
  - ♥ Say aloud: *I forgive, and I release this challenge with love. *Inhale, Exhale**
- ∞ SUPPORT: I felt supported today by/when _____
  _____
- ∞ GRATITUDE: I am grateful for _____
  _____
- ∞ INTENTION: My intention for the morning is _____

Tuesday

Morning PEP TALK

- ∞ In the mirror, with one hand on your heart: I LOVE YOU. YOU'VE GOT THIS, _____!
  (NAME)
- ∞ Affirmation: I (AM) _____
- ∞ I am grateful for (3+) _____
  _____
- ∞ I thank my body for _____
- ∞ HABIT TRACKER, Day ___ of 30

Wellbeing ACTIONS

- ☐ Today, I GET to _____ for me (prompts: JOY-FULL List p.15)
- ☐ Today, I GET to _____ my baby.
- ☐ Today, I GET to _____ for/with _____
  (e.g., spouse, kids, friends)

Nighttime REFLECTION

- ∞ WIN: I am _Celebrating_ myself for _____
- ∞ CHALLENGE: It felt hard when _____
  - ♥ I choose to see this as an opportunity to _____
  - ♥ Say aloud: *I forgive, and I release this challenge with love. *Inhale, Exhale**
- ∞ SUPPORT: I felt supported today by/when _____
  _____
- ∞ GRATITUDE: I am grateful for _____
  _____
- ∞ INTENTION: My intention for the morning is _____

Wednesday

Morning PEP TALK

- ∞ In the mirror, with one hand on your heart: I LOVE YOU. YOU'VE GOT THIS, _____!
  (NAME)
- ∞ Affirmation: I (AM) _____
- ∞ I am grateful for (3+) _____
  _____
- ∞ I thank my body for _____
- ∞ HABIT TRACKER, Day ___ of 30

Wellbeing ACTIONS

- ☐ Today, I GET to _____ for me (prompts: JOY-FULL List p.15)
- ☐ Today, I GET to _____ my baby.
- ☐ Today, I GET to _____ for/with _____
  (e.g., spouse, kids, friends)

Nighttime REFLECTION

- ∞ WIN: I am _Celebrating_ myself for _____
- ∞ CHALLENGE: It felt hard when _____
  - ♥ I choose to see this as an opportunity to _____
  - ♥ Say aloud: *I forgive, and I release this challenge with love.*
    Inhale, Exhale
- ∞ SUPPORT: I felt supported today by/when _____
  _____
- ∞ GRATITUDE: I am grateful for _____
  _____
- ∞ INTENTION: My intention for the morning is _____

Thursday

Morning PEP TALK

- ∞ In the mirror, with one hand on your heart: I LOVE YOU. YOU'VE GOT THIS, _____!
  (NAME)
- ∞ Affirmation: I (AM) _____
- ∞ I am grateful for (3+) _____
- ∞ I thank my body for _____
- ∞ HABIT TRACKER, Day ___ of 30

Wellbeing ACTIONS

- ☐ Today, I GET to _____ for me (prompts: JOY-FULL List p.15)
- ☐ Today, I GET to _____ my baby.
- ☐ Today, I GET to _____ for/with _____
  (e.g., spouse, kids, friends)

Nighttime REFLECTION

- ∞ WIN: I am *Celebrating* myself for _____
- ∞ CHALLENGE: It felt hard when _____
  - ♥ I choose to see this as an opportunity to _____
  - ♥ Say aloud: *I forgive, and I release this challenge with love. *Inhale, Exhale**
- ∞ SUPPORT: I felt supported today by/when _____
- ∞ GRATITUDE: I am grateful for _____
- ∞ INTENTION: My intention for the morning is _____

Friday

Morning PEP TALK

- ∞ In the mirror, with one hand on your heart: I LOVE YOU. YOU'VE GOT THIS, _____!
  _(NAME)
- ∞ Affirmation: I (AM) _____
- ∞ I am grateful for (3+) _____
  _____
- ∞ I thank my body for _____
- ∞ HABIT TRACKER, Day ___ of 30

Wellbeing ACTIONS

- ☐ Today, I GET to _____ for me _(prompts: JOY-FULL List p.15)
- ☐ Today, I GET to _____ my baby.
- ☐ Today, I GET to _____ for/with _____
  _(e.g., spouse, kids, friends)

Nighttime REFLECTION

- ∞ WIN: I am <u>*Celebrating*</u> myself for _____
- ∞ CHALLENGE: It felt hard when _____
  - ♥ I choose to see this as an opportunity to _____
  - ♥ Say aloud: *I forgive, and I release this challenge with love. *Inhale, Exhale**
- ∞ SUPPORT: I felt supported today by/when _____
  _____
- ∞ GRATITUDE: I am grateful for _____
  _____
- ∞ INTENTION: My intention for the morning is _____

Saturday

Morning PEP TALK

- ∞ In the mirror, with one hand on your heart: I LOVE YOU. YOU'VE GOT THIS, _____!
  (NAME)
- ∞ Affirmation: I (AM) _____
- ∞ I am grateful for (3+) _____
  _____
- ∞ I thank my body for _____
- ∞ HABIT TRACKER, Day ___ of 30

Wellbeing ACTIONS

- ☐ Today, I GET to _____ for me (prompts: JOY-FULL List p.15)
- ☐ Today, I GET to _____ my baby.
- ☐ Today, I GET to _____ for/with _____
  (e.g., spouse, kids, friends)

Nighttime REFLECTION

- ∞ WIN: I am *Celebrating* myself for _____
- ∞ CHALLENGE: It felt hard when _____
  - ♥ I choose to see this as an opportunity to _____
  - ♥ Say aloud: *I forgive, and I release this challenge with love.* *Inhale, Exhale*
- ∞ SUPPORT: I felt supported today by/when _____
  _____
- ∞ GRATITUDE: I am grateful for _____
  _____
- ∞ INTENTION: My intention for the morning is _____

Sunday

Morning PEP TALK

- ∞ In the mirror, with one hand on your heart: I LOVE YOU. YOU'VE GOT THIS, _____!
   (NAME)
- ∞ Affirmation: I (AM) _____
- ∞ I am grateful for (3+) _____
  _____
- ∞ I thank my body for _____
- ∞ HABIT TRACKER, Day ___ of 30

Wellbeing ACTIONS

- ☐ Today, I GET to _____ for me (prompts: JOY-FULL List p.15)
- ☐ Today, I GET to _____ my baby.
- ☐ Today, I GET to _____ for/with _____
   (e.g., spouse, kids, friends)

Nighttime REFLECTION

- ∞ WIN: I am *Celebrating* myself for _____
- ∞ CHALLENGE: It felt hard when _____
   - ♥ I choose to see this as an opportunity to _____
   - ♥ Say aloud: *I forgive, and I release this challenge with love. *Inhale, Exhale**
- ∞ SUPPORT: I felt supported today by/when _____
  _____
- ∞ GRATITUDE: I am grateful for _____
  _____
- ∞ INTENTION: My intention for the morning is _____

What's happening this week

Week of: _____

- ♥ Affirmation: I _____

- ♥ I will show myself grace this week by _____

- ♥ I am looking forward to _____

- ♥ I get to ask for support with _____

    By (action step) _____

- ☐ Review #2-6 from the Monthly Wellbeing Check-in. Take a moment to visualize yourself integrating these feelings, actions, and thoughts now, as well as throughout this week.

- ☐ Review upcoming appointments and set an alarm in your phone as needed.

Grocery list:
(TIP: Record here and take a picture to bring ease to the next grocery store trip.)

_____	_____	_____
_____	_____	_____
_____	_____	_____
_____	_____	_____
_____	_____	_____
_____	_____	_____
_____	_____	_____
_____	_____	_____

Monday

Morning PEP TALK

- ∞ In the mirror, with one hand on your heart: I LOVE YOU. YOU'VE GOT THIS, _____!
  (NAME)
- ∞ Affirmation: I (AM) _____
- ∞ I am grateful for (3+) _____
  _____
- ∞ I thank my body for _____
- ∞ HABIT TRACKER, Day ___ of 30

Wellbeing ACTIONS

- ☐ Today, I GET to _____ for me (prompts: JOY-FULL List p.15)
- ☐ Today, I GET to _____ my baby.
- ☐ Today, I GET to _____ for/with _____
  (e.g., spouse, kids, friends)

Nighttime REFLECTION

- ∞ WIN: I am *Celebrating* myself for _____
- ∞ CHALLENGE: It felt hard when _____
  - ♥ I choose to see this as an opportunity to _____
  - ♥ Say aloud: *I forgive, and I release this challenge with love.* *Inhale, Exhale*
- ∞ SUPPORT: I felt supported today by/when _____
  _____
- ∞ GRATITUDE: I am grateful for _____
  _____
- ∞ INTENTION: My intention for the morning is _____

Tuesday

Morning PEP TALK

- ∞ In the mirror, with one hand on your heart: I LOVE YOU. YOU'VE GOT THIS, _____!
  (NAME)
- ∞ Affirmation: I (AM) _____
- ∞ I am grateful for (3+) _____
  _____
- ∞ I thank my body for _____
- ∞ HABIT TRACKER, Day ___ of 30

Wellbeing ACTIONS

- ☐ Today, I GET to _____ for me (prompts: JOY-FULL List p.15)
- ☐ Today, I GET to _____ my baby.
- ☐ Today, I GET to _____ for/with _____
  (e.g., spouse, kids, friends)

Nighttime REFLECTION

- ∞ WIN: I am *Celebrating* myself for _____
- ∞ CHALLENGE: It felt hard when _____
  - ♥ I choose to see this as an opportunity to _____
  - ♥ Say aloud: *I forgive, and I release this challenge with love.* *Inhale, Exhale*
- ∞ SUPPORT: I felt supported today by/when _____
  _____
- ∞ GRATITUDE: I am grateful for _____
  _____
- ∞ INTENTION: My intention for the morning is _____

Wednesday

Morning PEP TALK

- ∞ In the mirror, with one hand on your heart: I LOVE YOU. YOU'VE GOT THIS, _____!
  (NAME)
- ∞ Affirmation: I (AM) _____
- ∞ I am grateful for (3+) _____
  _____
- ∞ I thank my body for _____
- ∞ HABIT TRACKER, Day ___ of 30

Wellbeing ACTIONS

- ☐ Today, I GET to _____ for me (prompts: JOY-FULL List p.15)
- ☐ Today, I GET to _____ my baby.
- ☐ Today, I GET to _____ for/with _____
  (e.g., spouse, kids, friends)

Nighttime REFLECTION

- ∞ WIN: I am _Celebrating_ myself for _____
- ∞ CHALLENGE: It felt hard when _____
  - ♥ I choose to see this as an opportunity to _____
  - ♥ Say aloud: *I forgive, and I release this challenge with love. *Inhale, Exhale**
- ∞ SUPPORT: I felt supported today by/when _____
  _____
- ∞ GRATITUDE: I am grateful for _____
  _____
- ∞ INTENTION: My intention for the morning is _____

Thursday

Morning PEP TALK

- ∞ In the mirror, with one hand on your heart: I LOVE YOU. YOU'VE GOT THIS, _____!
  (NAME)
- ∞ Affirmation: I (AM) _____
- ∞ I am grateful for (3+) _____
  _____
- ∞ I thank my body for _____
- ∞ HABIT TRACKER, Day ___ of 30

Wellbeing ACTIONS

- ☐ Today, I GET to _____ for me (prompts: JOY-FULL List p.15)
- ☐ Today, I GET to _____ my baby.
- ☐ Today, I GET to _____ for/with _____
  (e.g., spouse, kids, friends)

Nighttime REFLECTION

- ∞ WIN: I am *Celebrating* myself for _____
- ∞ CHALLENGE: It felt hard when _____
  - ♥ I choose to see this as an opportunity to _____
  - ♥ Say aloud: *I forgive, and I release this challenge with love. *Inhale, Exhale**
- ∞ SUPPORT: I felt supported today by/when _____
  _____
- ∞ GRATITUDE: I am grateful for _____
  _____
- ∞ INTENTION: My intention for the morning is _____

Friday

Morning PEP TALK

- ∞ In the mirror, with one hand on your heart: I LOVE YOU. YOU'VE GOT THIS, _____!
  (NAME)
- ∞ Affirmation: I (AM) _____
- ∞ I am grateful for (3+) _____
  _____
- ∞ I thank my body for _____
- ∞ HABIT TRACKER, Day ___ of 30

Wellbeing ACTIONS

- ☐ Today, I GET to _____ for me (prompts: JOY-FULL List p.15)
- ☐ Today, I GET to _____ my baby.
- ☐ Today, I GET to _____ for/with _____
  (e.g., spouse, kids, friends)

Nighttime REFLECTION

- ∞ WIN: I am _Celebrating_ myself for _____
- ∞ CHALLENGE: It felt hard when _____
  - ♥ I choose to see this as an opportunity to _____
  - ♥ Say aloud: *I forgive, and I release this challenge with love. *Inhale, Exhale**
- ∞ SUPPORT: I felt supported today by/when _____
  _____
- ∞ GRATITUDE: I am grateful for _____
  _____
- ∞ INTENTION: My intention for the morning is _____

Saturday

Morning PEP TALK

- ∞ In the mirror, with one hand on your heart: I LOVE YOU. YOU'VE GOT THIS, _____!
  (NAME)
- ∞ Affirmation: I (AM) _____
- ∞ I am grateful for (3+) _____
  _____
- ∞ I thank my body for _____
- ∞ HABIT TRACKER, Day ___ of 30

Wellbeing ACTIONS

- ☐ Today, I GET to _____ for me (prompts: JOY-FULL List p.15)
- ☐ Today, I GET to _____ my baby.
- ☐ Today, I GET to _____ for/with _____
  (e.g., spouse, kids, friends)

Nighttime REFLECTION

- ∞ WIN: I am _Celebrating_ myself for _____
- ∞ CHALLENGE: It felt hard when _____
  - ♥ I choose to see this as an opportunity to _____
  - ♥ Say aloud: *I forgive, and I release this challenge with love. *Inhale, Exhale**
- ∞ SUPPORT: I felt supported today by/when _____
  _____
- ∞ GRATITUDE: I am grateful for _____
  _____
- ∞ INTENTION: My intention for the morning is _____

Sunday

Morning PEP TALK

- ∞ In the mirror, with one hand on your heart: I LOVE YOU. YOU'VE GOT THIS, _____!
  (NAME)
- ∞ Affirmation: I (AM) _____
- ∞ I am grateful for (3+) _____
  _____
- ∞ I thank my body for _____
- ∞ HABIT TRACKER, Day ___ of 30

Wellbeing ACTIONS

- ☐ Today, I GET to _____ for me (prompts: JOY-FULL List p.15)
- ☐ Today, I GET to _____ my baby.
- ☐ Today, I GET to _____ for/with _____
  (e.g., spouse, kids, friends)

Nighttime REFLECTION

- ∞ WIN: I am *Celebrating* myself for _____
- ∞ CHALLENGE: It felt hard when _____
  - ♥ I choose to see this as an opportunity to _____
  - ♥ Say aloud: *I forgive, and I release this challenge with love.*
    Inhale, Exhale
- ∞ SUPPORT: I felt supported today by/when _____
  _____
- ∞ GRATITUDE: I am grateful for _____
  _____
- ∞ INTENTION: My intention for the morning is _____

What's happening this week

Week of: _____

- ♥ Affirmation: I _____
- ♥ I will show myself grace this week by _____
- ♥ I am looking forward to _____
- ♥ I get to ask for support with _____

    By (action step) _____

- ☐ Review #2-6 from the Monthly Wellbeing Check-in. Take a moment to visualize yourself integrating these feelings, actions, and thoughts now, as well as throughout this week.

- ☐ Review upcoming appointments and set an alarm in your phone as needed.

Grocery list:
(TIP: Record here and take a picture to bring ease to the next grocery store trip.)

_____   _____   _____

_____   _____   _____

_____   _____   _____

_____   _____   _____

_____   _____   _____

_____   _____   _____

_____   _____   _____

Monday

Morning PEP TALK

- ∞ In the mirror, with one hand on your heart: I LOVE YOU. YOU'VE GOT THIS, _____!
  (NAME)
- ∞ Affirmation: I (AM) _____
- ∞ I am grateful for (3+) _____
  _____
- ∞ I thank my body for _____
- ∞ HABIT TRACKER, Day ___ of 30

Wellbeing ACTIONS

- ☐ Today, I GET to _____ for me (prompts: JOY-FULL List p.15)
- ☐ Today, I GET to _____ my baby.
- ☐ Today, I GET to _____ for/with _____
  (e.g., spouse, kids, friends)

Nighttime REFLECTION

- ∞ WIN: I am *Celebrating* myself for _____
- ∞ CHALLENGE: It felt hard when _____
  - ♥ I choose to see this as an opportunity to _____
  - ♥ Say aloud: *I forgive, and I release this challenge with love. *Inhale, Exhale**
- ∞ SUPPORT: I felt supported today by/when _____
  _____
- ∞ GRATITUDE: I am grateful for _____
  _____
- ∞ INTENTION: My intention for the morning is _____

Tuesday

Morning PEP TALK

- ∞ In the mirror, with one hand on your heart: I LOVE YOU. YOU'VE GOT THIS, _____!
  (NAME)
- ∞ Affirmation: I (AM) _____
- ∞ I am grateful for (3+) _____
  _____
- ∞ I thank my body for _____
- ∞ HABIT TRACKER, Day ___ of 30

Wellbeing ACTIONS

- ☐ Today, I GET to _____ for me (prompts: JOY-FULL List p.15)
- ☐ Today, I GET to _____ my baby.
- ☐ Today, I GET to _____ for/with _____
  (e.g., spouse, kids, friends)

Nighttime REFLECTION

- ∞ WIN: I am <u>Celebrating</u> myself for _____
- ∞ CHALLENGE: It felt hard when _____
  - ♥ I choose to see this as an opportunity to _____
  - ♥ Say aloud: *I forgive, and I release this challenge with love.* *Inhale, Exhale*
- ∞ SUPPORT: I felt supported today by/when _____
  _____
- ∞ GRATITUDE: I am grateful for _____
  _____
- ∞ INTENTION: My intention for the morning is _____

Wednesday

Morning PEP TALK

- ∞ In the mirror, with one hand on your heart: I LOVE YOU. YOU'VE GOT THIS, _____!

(NAME)
- ∞ Affirmation: I (AM) _____
- ∞ I am grateful for (3+) _____
  _____
- ∞ I thank my body for _____
- ∞ HABIT TRACKER, Day ___ of 30

Wellbeing ACTIONS

- ☐ Today, I GET to _____ for me (prompts: JOY-FULL List p.15)
- ☐ Today, I GET to _____ my baby.
- ☐ Today, I GET to _____ for/with _____

(e.g., spouse, kids, friends)

Nighttime REFLECTION

- ∞ WIN: I am _Celebrating_ myself for _____
- ∞ CHALLENGE: It felt hard when _____
  - ♥ I choose to see this as an opportunity to _____
  - ♥ Say aloud: *I forgive, and I release this challenge with love. *Inhale, Exhale**
- ∞ SUPPORT: I felt supported today by/when _____
  _____
- ∞ GRATITUDE: I am grateful for _____
  _____
- ∞ INTENTION: My intention for the morning is _____

Thursday

Morning PEP TALK

- ∞ In the mirror, with one hand on your heart: I LOVE YOU. YOU'VE GOT THIS, _____ !
  (NAME)
- ∞ Affirmation: I (AM) _____
- ∞ I am grateful for (3+) _____
   _____
- ∞ I thank my body for _____
- ∞ HABIT TRACKER, Day ___ of 30

Wellbeing ACTIONS

- ☐ Today, I GET to _____ for me (prompts: JOY-FULL List p.15)
- ☐ Today, I GET to _____ my baby.
- ☐ Today, I GET to _____ for/with _____
  (e.g., spouse, kids, friends)

Nighttime REFLECTION

- ∞ WIN: I am _Celebrating_ myself for _____
- ∞ CHALLENGE: It felt hard when _____
  - ♥ I choose to see this as an opportunity to _____
  - ♥ Say aloud: _I forgive, and I release this challenge with love._ *Inhale, Exhale*
- ∞ SUPPORT: I felt supported today by/when _____
  _____
- ∞ GRATITUDE: I am grateful for _____
  _____
- ∞ INTENTION: My intention for the morning is _____

Friday

Morning PEP TALK

- ∞ In the mirror, with one hand on your heart: I LOVE YOU. YOU'VE GOT THIS, _____!

(NAME)
- ∞ Affirmation: I (AM) _____
- ∞ I am grateful for (3+) _____
  _____
- ∞ I thank my body for _____
- ∞ HABIT TRACKER, Day ___ of 30

Wellbeing ACTIONS

- ☐ Today, I GET to _____ for me (prompts: JOY-FULL List p.15)
- ☐ Today, I GET to _____ my baby.
- ☐ Today, I GET to _____ for/with _____

(e.g., spouse, kids, friends)

Nighttime REFLECTION

- ∞ WIN: I am *Celebrating* myself for _____
- ∞ CHALLENGE: It felt hard when _____
  - ♥ I choose to see this as an opportunity to _____
  - ♥ Say aloud: *I forgive, and I release this challenge with love. *Inhale, Exhale**
- ∞ SUPPORT: I felt supported today by/when _____
  _____
- ∞ GRATITUDE: I am grateful for _____
  _____
- ∞ INTENTION: My intention for the morning is _____

Saturday

Morning PEP TALK

- ∞ In the mirror, with one hand on your heart: I LOVE YOU. YOU'VE GOT THIS, _____!
  (NAME)
- ∞ Affirmation: I (AM) _____
- ∞ I am grateful for (3+) _____
  _____
- ∞ I thank my body for _____
- ∞ HABIT TRACKER, Day ___ of 30

Wellbeing ACTIONS

- ☐ Today, I GET to _____ for me (prompts: JOY-FULL List p.15)
- ☐ Today, I GET to _____ my baby.
- ☐ Today, I GET to _____ for/with _____
  (e.g., spouse, kids, friends)

Nighttime REFLECTION

- ∞ WIN: I am *Celebrating* myself for _____
- ∞ CHALLENGE: It felt hard when _____
  - ♥ I choose to see this as an opportunity to _____
  - ♥ Say aloud: *I forgive, and I release this challenge with love. *Inhale, Exhale**
- ∞ SUPPORT: I felt supported today by/when _____
  _____
- ∞ GRATITUDE: I am grateful for _____
  _____
- ∞ INTENTION: My intention for the morning is _____

Sunday

Morning PEP TALK

- ∞ In the mirror, with one hand on your heart: I LOVE YOU. YOU'VE GOT THIS, _____!
  (NAME)
- ∞ Affirmation: I (AM) _____
- ∞ I am grateful for (3+) _____
  _____
- ∞ I thank my body for _____
- ∞ HABIT TRACKER, Day ___ of 30

Wellbeing ACTIONS

- ☐ Today, I GET to _____ for me (prompts: JOY-FULL List p.15)
- ☐ Today, I GET to _____ my baby.
- ☐ Today, I GET to _____ for/with _____
  (e.g., spouse, kids, friends)

Nighttime REFLECTION

- ∞ WIN: I am *Celebrating* myself for _____
- ∞ CHALLENGE: It felt hard when _____
  - ♥ I choose to see this as an opportunity to _____
  - ♥ Say aloud: *I forgive, and I release this challenge with love.*
    Inhale, Exhale
- ∞ SUPPORT: I felt supported today by/when _____
  _____
- ∞ GRATITUDE: I am grateful for _____
  _____
- ∞ INTENTION: My intention for the morning is _____

Monthly Recap

- I am Celebrating _____!
    - In my head, I feel _____
    - In my heart, I feel _____
    - In my body, I feel _____
- My favourite activities this month were _____
  _____
    because _____
- My favourite affirmations this month were _____
  _____
    because _____
- It felt hard when _____
    From this, I learned _____
- I feel more joy and ease in my life when I _____
  _____
- I felt most supported this month when _____
- I am grateful for _____
- The boundary I set up at the beginning of the month helped me by
  _____
- I am celebrating my new habit this month!
    I am bringing this new habit with me into next month because (impact)
    _____
- Special milestones/memories (date and event):

MONTH:

Free write/Notes/Lessons/Draw

MONTH: _____

SUNDAY	MONDAY	TUESDAY	WEDNESDAY
___	___	___	___
___	___	___	___
___	___	___	___
___	___	___	___
___	___	___	___

Record special dates, appointments, milestones, etc.

THURSDAY	FRIDAY	SATURDAY	NOTES
____	____	____	
____	____	____	
____	____	____	
____	____	____	
____	____	____	

Monthly Wellbeing Check-in

MONTH: _____

1. How do I feel right now?

    ◊   In my head (mentally): _____

    _____

    ◊   In my heart (emotionally): _____

    _____

    ◊   In my body (physically): _____

    _____

2. How do I desire to feel?

    ◊   In my head (mentally): _____

    _____

    ◊   In my heart (emotionally): _____

    _____

    ◊   In my body (physically): _____

    _____

3. What actions can I take to help me feel the way I described above? What thoughts can I have to help me feel this way?

    ◊   In my head (mentally): _____

    _____

    ◊   In my heart (emotionally): _____

    _____

    ◊   In my body (physically): _____

    _____

4. What am I excited for this month? _____

_____

5. What boundary am I setting up this month? _____

_____

   ◊   Action(s) to set up this boundary: _____

       _____

6. HABIT TRACKER (e.g., action/thought you wrote about for your desired feeling in #3):

I _____ am developing the habit of _____ this month.
　(NAME)

Picture this as a habit already. How do I feel? How am I showing up? What is different?

_____

_____

_____

_____

_____

_____

I understand that I may miss a day. I will show myself grace and re-commit the next day.

This habit supports me.

I am doing my best and I am Thriving!

What's happening this week

Week of: _____

- ♥ Affirmation: I _____

- ♥ I will show myself grace this week by _____

- ♥ I am looking forward to _____

- ♥ I get to ask for support with _____

   By (action step) _____

- ☐ Review #2-6 from the Monthly Wellbeing Check-in. Take a moment to visualize yourself integrating these feelings, actions, and thoughts now, as well as throughout this week.

- ☐ Review upcoming appointments and set an alarm in your phone as needed.

Grocery list:
(TIP: Record here and take a picture to bring ease to the next grocery store trip.)

_____	_____	_____
_____	_____	_____
_____	_____	_____
_____	_____	_____
_____	_____	_____
_____	_____	_____
_____	_____	_____

Monday

Morning PEP TALK

- ∞ In the mirror, with one hand on your heart: I LOVE YOU. YOU'VE GOT THIS, _____!
  (NAME)
- ∞ Affirmation: I (AM) _____
- ∞ I am grateful for (3+) _____
  _____
- ∞ I thank my body for _____
- ∞ HABIT TRACKER, Day ___ of 30

Wellbeing ACTIONS

- ☐ Today, I GET to _____ for me (prompts: JOY-FULL List p.15)
- ☐ Today, I GET to _____ my baby.
- ☐ Today, I GET to _____ for/with _____
  (e.g., spouse, kids, friends)

Nighttime REFLECTION

- ∞ WIN: I am *Celebrating* myself for _____
- ∞ CHALLENGE: It felt hard when _____
  - ♥ I choose to see this as an opportunity to _____
  - ♥ Say aloud: *I forgive, and I release this challenge with love. *Inhale, Exhale**
- ∞ SUPPORT: I felt supported today by/when _____
  _____
- ∞ GRATITUDE: I am grateful for _____
  _____
- ∞ INTENTION: My intention for the morning is _____

Tuesday

Morning PEP TALK

- ∞ In the mirror, with one hand on your heart: I LOVE YOU. YOU'VE GOT THIS, _____!
  (NAME)
- ∞ Affirmation: I (AM) _____
- ∞ I am grateful for (3+) _____
  _____
- ∞ I thank my body for _____
- ∞ HABIT TRACKER, Day ___ of 30

Wellbeing ACTIONS

- ☐ Today, I GET to _____ for me (prompts: JOY-FULL List p.15)
- ☐ Today, I GET to _____ my baby.
- ☐ Today, I GET to _____ for/with _____
  (e.g., spouse, kids, friends)

Nighttime REFLECTION

- ∞ WIN: I am _Celebrating_ myself for _____
- ∞ CHALLENGE: It felt hard when _____
  - ♥ I choose to see this as an opportunity to _____
  - ♥ Say aloud: *I forgive, and I release this challenge with love.* *Inhale, Exhale*
- ∞ SUPPORT: I felt supported today by/when _____
  _____
- ∞ GRATITUDE: I am grateful for _____
  _____
- ∞ INTENTION: My intention for the morning is _____

Wednesday

Morning PEP TALK

- ∞ In the mirror, with one hand on your heart: I LOVE YOU. YOU'VE GOT THIS, _____!
  (NAME)
- ∞ Affirmation: I (AM) _____
- ∞ I am grateful for (3+) _____
  _____
- ∞ I thank my body for _____
- ∞ HABIT TRACKER, Day ___ of 30

Wellbeing ACTIONS

- ☐ Today, I GET to _____ for me (prompts: JOY-FULL List p.15)
- ☐ Today, I GET to _____ my baby.
- ☐ Today, I GET to _____ for/with _____
  (e.g., spouse, kids, friends)

Nighttime REFLECTION

- ∞ WIN: I am *Celebrating* myself for _____
- ∞ CHALLENGE: It felt hard when _____
  - ♥ I choose to see this as an opportunity to _____
  - ♥ Say aloud: *I forgive, and I release this challenge with love. *Inhale, Exhale**
- ∞ SUPPORT: I felt supported today by/when _____
  _____
- ∞ GRATITUDE: I am grateful for _____
  _____
- ∞ INTENTION: My intention for the morning is _____

Thursday

Morning PEP TALK

- ∞ In the mirror, with one hand on your heart: I LOVE YOU. YOU'VE GOT THIS, _____!

(NAME)
- ∞ Affirmation: I (AM) _____
- ∞ I am grateful for (3+) _____
  _____
- ∞ I thank my body for _____
- ∞ HABIT TRACKER, Day ___ of 30

Wellbeing ACTIONS

- ☐ Today, I GET to _____ for me (prompts: JOY-FULL List p.15)
- ☐ Today, I GET to _____ my baby.
- ☐ Today, I GET to _____ for/with _____

(e.g., spouse, kids, friends)

Nighttime REFLECTION

- ∞ WIN: I am *Celebrating* myself for _____
- ∞ CHALLENGE: It felt hard when _____
    - ♥ I choose to see this as an opportunity to _____
    - ♥ Say aloud: *I forgive, and I release this challenge with love. *Inhale, Exhale**
- ∞ SUPPORT: I felt supported today by/when _____
  _____
- ∞ GRATITUDE: I am grateful for _____
  _____
- ∞ INTENTION: My intention for the morning is _____

Friday

Morning PEP TALK

- ∞ In the mirror, with one hand on your heart: I LOVE YOU. YOU'VE GOT THIS, _____!
  (NAME)
- ∞ Affirmation: I (AM) _____
- ∞ I am grateful for (3+) _____
  _____
- ∞ I thank my body for _____
- ∞ HABIT TRACKER, Day ___ of 30

Wellbeing ACTIONS

- ☐ Today, I GET to _____ for me (prompts: JOY-FULL List p.15)
- ☐ Today, I GET to _____ my baby.
- ☐ Today, I GET to _____ for/with _____
  (e.g., spouse, kids, friends)

Nighttime REFLECTION

- ∞ WIN: I am *Celebrating* myself for _____
- ∞ CHALLENGE: It felt hard when _____
  - ♥ I choose to see this as an opportunity to _____
  - ♥ Say aloud: *I forgive, and I release this challenge with love.*
    Inhale, Exhale
- ∞ SUPPORT: I felt supported today by/when _____
  _____
- ∞ GRATITUDE: I am grateful for _____
  _____
- ∞ INTENTION: My intention for the morning is _____

Saturday

Morning PEP TALK

- ∞ In the mirror, with one hand on your heart: I LOVE YOU. YOU'VE GOT THIS, _____!
  (NAME)
- ∞ Affirmation: I (AM) _____
- ∞ I am grateful for (3+) _____
  _____
- ∞ I thank my body for _____
- ∞ HABIT TRACKER, Day ___ of 30

Wellbeing ACTIONS

- ☐ Today, I GET to _____ for me (prompts: JOY-FULL List p.15)
- ☐ Today, I GET to _____ my baby.
- ☐ Today, I GET to _____ for/with _____
  (e.g., spouse, kids, friends)

Nighttime REFLECTION

- ∞ WIN: I am <u>Celebrating</u> myself for _____
- ∞ CHALLENGE: It felt hard when _____
  - ♥ I choose to see this as an opportunity to _____
  - ♥ Say aloud: *I forgive, and I release this challenge with love. *Inhale, Exhale**
- ∞ SUPPORT: I felt supported today by/when _____
  _____
- ∞ GRATITUDE: I am grateful for _____
  _____
- ∞ INTENTION: My intention for the morning is _____

Sunday

Morning PEP TALK

- ∞ In the mirror, with one hand on your heart: I LOVE YOU. YOU'VE GOT THIS, _____!
  (NAME)
- ∞ Affirmation: I (AM) _____
- ∞ I am grateful for (3+) _____
  _____
- ∞ I thank my body for _____
- ∞ HABIT TRACKER, Day ___ of 30

Wellbeing ACTIONS

- ☐ Today, I GET to _____ for me (prompts: JOY-FULL List p.15)
- ☐ Today, I GET to _____ my baby.
- ☐ Today, I GET to _____ for/with _____
  (e.g., spouse, kids, friends)

Nighttime REFLECTION

- ∞ WIN: I am *Celebrating* myself for _____
- ∞ CHALLENGE: It felt hard when _____
  - ♥ I choose to see this as an opportunity to _____
  - ♥ Say aloud: *I forgive, and I release this challenge with love.* *Inhale, Exhale*
- ∞ SUPPORT: I felt supported today by/when _____
  _____
- ∞ GRATITUDE: I am grateful for _____
  _____
- ∞ INTENTION: My intention for the morning is _____

What's happening this week

Week of: _____

- ♥ Affirmation: I _____

- ♥ I will show myself grace this week by _____

- ♥ I am looking forward to _____

- ♥ I get to ask for support with _____

    By (action step) _____

- ☐ Review #2-6 from the Monthly Wellbeing Check-in. Take a moment to visualize yourself integrating these feelings, actions, and thoughts now, as well as throughout this week.

- ☐ Review upcoming appointments and set an alarm in your phone as needed.

Grocery list:
(TIP: Record here and take a picture to bring ease to the next grocery store trip.)

_____   _____   _____

_____   _____   _____

_____   _____   _____

_____   _____   _____

_____   _____   _____

_____   _____   _____

_____   _____   _____

Monday

Morning PEP TALK

- ∞ In the mirror, with one hand on your heart: I LOVE YOU. YOU'VE GOT THIS, _____!
  (NAME)
- ∞ Affirmation: I (AM) _____
- ∞ I am grateful for (3+) _____
  _____
- ∞ I thank my body for _____
- ∞ HABIT TRACKER, Day ___ of 30

Wellbeing ACTIONS

- ☐ Today, I GET to _____ for me (prompts: JOY-FULL List p.15)
- ☐ Today, I GET to _____ my baby.
- ☐ Today, I GET to _____ for/with _____
  (e.g., spouse, kids, friends)

Nighttime REFLECTION

- ∞ WIN: I am *Celebrating* myself for _____
- ∞ CHALLENGE: It felt hard when _____
  - ♥ I choose to see this as an opportunity to _____
  - ♥ Say aloud: *I forgive, and I release this challenge with love. *Inhale, Exhale**
- ∞ SUPPORT: I felt supported today by/when _____
  _____
- ∞ GRATITUDE: I am grateful for _____
  _____
- ∞ INTENTION: My intention for the morning is _____

Tuesday

Morning PEP TALK

- ∞ In the mirror, with one hand on your heart: I LOVE YOU. YOU'VE GOT THIS, _____!
  (NAME)
- ∞ Affirmation: I (AM) _____
- ∞ I am grateful for (3+) _____
  _____
- ∞ I thank my body for _____
- ∞ HABIT TRACKER, Day ___ of 30

Wellbeing ACTIONS

- ☐ Today, I GET to _____ for me (prompts: JOY-FULL List p.15)
- ☐ Today, I GET to _____ my baby.
- ☐ Today, I GET to _____ for/with _____
  (e.g., spouse, kids, friends)

Nighttime REFLECTION

- ∞ WIN: I am *Celebrating* myself for _____
- ∞ CHALLENGE: It felt hard when _____
  - ♥ I choose to see this as an opportunity to _____
  - ♥ Say aloud: *I forgive, and I release this challenge with love. *Inhale, Exhale**
- ∞ SUPPORT: I felt supported today by/when _____
  _____
- ∞ GRATITUDE: I am grateful for _____
  _____
- ∞ INTENTION: My intention for the morning is _____

Wednesday

Morning PEP TALK

- ∞ In the mirror, with one hand on your heart: I LOVE YOU. YOU'VE GOT THIS, _____!
  (NAME)
- ∞ Affirmation: I (AM) _____
- ∞ I am grateful for (3+) _____
  _____
- ∞ I thank my body for _____
- ∞ HABIT TRACKER, Day ___ of 30

Wellbeing ACTIONS

- ☐ Today, I GET to _____ for me (prompts: JOY-FULL List p.15)
- ☐ Today, I GET to _____ my baby.
- ☐ Today, I GET to _____ for/with _____
  (e.g., spouse, kids, friends)

Nighttime REFLECTION

- ∞ WIN: I am *Celebrating* myself for _____
- ∞ CHALLENGE: It felt hard when _____
  - ♥ I choose to see this as an opportunity to _____
  - ♥ Say aloud: *I forgive, and I release this challenge with love. *Inhale, Exhale**
- ∞ SUPPORT: I felt supported today by/when _____
  _____
- ∞ GRATITUDE: I am grateful for _____
  _____
- ∞ INTENTION: My intention for the morning is _____

Thursday

Morning PEP TALK

- ∞ In the mirror, with one hand on your heart: I LOVE YOU. YOU'VE GOT THIS, _____!
  (NAME)
- ∞ Affirmation: I (AM) _____
- ∞ I am grateful for (3+) _____
  _____
- ∞ I thank my body for _____
- ∞ HABIT TRACKER, Day ___ of 30

Wellbeing ACTIONS

- ☐ Today, I GET to _____ for me (prompts: JOY-FULL List p.15)
- ☐ Today, I GET to _____ my baby.
- ☐ Today, I GET to _____ for/with _____
  (e.g., spouse, kids, friends)

Nighttime REFLECTION

- ∞ WIN: I am *Celebrating* myself for _____
- ∞ CHALLENGE: It felt hard when _____
  - ♥ I choose to see this as an opportunity to _____
  - ♥ Say aloud: *I forgive, and I release this challenge with love. *Inhale, Exhale**
- ∞ SUPPORT: I felt supported today by/when _____
  _____
- ∞ GRATITUDE: I am grateful for _____
  _____
- ∞ INTENTION: My intention for the morning is _____

Friday

Morning PEP TALK

- ∞ In the mirror, with one hand on your heart: I LOVE YOU. YOU'VE GOT THIS, _____!
  (NAME)
- ∞ Affirmation: I (AM) _____
- ∞ I am grateful for (3+) _____
  _____
- ∞ I thank my body for _____
- ∞ HABIT TRACKER, Day ___ of 30

Wellbeing ACTIONS

- ☐ Today, I GET to _____ for me (prompts: JOY-FULL List p.15)
- ☐ Today, I GET to _____ my baby.
- ☐ Today, I GET to _____ for/with _____
  (e.g., spouse, kids, friends)

Nighttime REFLECTION

- ∞ WIN: I am _Celebrating_ myself for _____
- ∞ CHALLENGE: It felt hard when _____
  - ♥ I choose to see this as an opportunity to _____
  - ♥ Say aloud: *I forgive, and I release this challenge with love.* *Inhale, Exhale*
- ∞ SUPPORT: I felt supported today by/when _____
  _____
- ∞ GRATITUDE: I am grateful for _____
  _____
- ∞ INTENTION: My intention for the morning is _____

Saturday

Morning PEP TALK

- ∞ In the mirror, with one hand on your heart: I LOVE YOU. YOU'VE GOT THIS, _____!
  (NAME)
- ∞ Affirmation: I (AM) _____
- ∞ I am grateful for (3+) _____
- ∞ I thank my body for _____
- ∞ HABIT TRACKER, Day ___ of 30

Wellbeing ACTIONS

- ☐ Today, I GET to _____ for me (prompts: JOY-FULL List p.15)
- ☐ Today, I GET to _____ my baby.
- ☐ Today, I GET to _____ for/with _____
  (e.g., spouse, kids, friends)

Nighttime REFLECTION

- ∞ WIN: I am *Celebrating* myself for _____
- ∞ CHALLENGE: It felt hard when _____
  - ♥ I choose to see this as an opportunity to _____
  - ♥ Say aloud: *I forgive, and I release this challenge with love. *Inhale, Exhale**
- ∞ SUPPORT: I felt supported today by/when _____
- ∞ GRATITUDE: I am grateful for _____
- ∞ INTENTION: My intention for the morning is _____

Sunday

Morning PEP TALK

- ∞ In the mirror, with one hand on your heart: I LOVE YOU. YOU'VE GOT THIS, _____!
  (NAME)
- ∞ Affirmation: I (AM) _____
- ∞ I am grateful for (3+) _____
  _____
- ∞ I thank my body for _____
- ∞ HABIT TRACKER, Day ___ of 30

Wellbeing ACTIONS

- ☐ Today, I GET to _____ for me (prompts: JOY-FULL List p.15)
- ☐ Today, I GET to _____ my baby.
- ☐ Today, I GET to _____ for/with _____
  (e.g., spouse, kids, friends)

Nighttime REFLECTION

- ∞ WIN: I am _Celebrating_ myself for _____
- ∞ CHALLENGE: It felt hard when _____
  - ♥ I choose to see this as an opportunity to _____
  - ♥ Say aloud: *I forgive, and I release this challenge with love.* *Inhale, Exhale*
- ∞ SUPPORT: I felt supported today by/when _____
  _____
- ∞ GRATITUDE: I am grateful for _____
  _____
- ∞ INTENTION: My intention for the morning is _____

What's happening this week

Week of: _____

- ♥ Affirmation: I _____

- ♥ I will show myself grace this week by _____

- ♥ I am looking forward to _____

- ♥ I get to ask for support with _____

    By (action step) _____

- ☐ Review #2-6 from the Monthly Wellbeing Check-in. Take a moment to visualize yourself integrating these feelings, actions, and thoughts now, as well as throughout this week.

- ☐ Review upcoming appointments and set an alarm in your phone as needed.

Grocery list:
(TIP: Record here and take a picture to bring ease to the next grocery store trip.)

_____	_____	_____
_____	_____	_____
_____	_____	_____
_____	_____	_____
_____	_____	_____
_____	_____	_____
_____	_____	_____
_____	_____	_____

Monday

Morning PEP TALK

- ∞ In the mirror, with one hand on your heart: I LOVE YOU. YOU'VE GOT THIS, _____!
  (NAME)
- ∞ Affirmation: I (AM) _____
- ∞ I am grateful for (3+) _____
  _____
- ∞ I thank my body for _____
- ∞ HABIT TRACKER, Day ___ of 30

Wellbeing ACTIONS

- ☐ Today, I GET to _____ for me (prompts: JOY-FULL List p.15)
- ☐ Today, I GET to _____ my baby.
- ☐ Today, I GET to _____ for/with _____
  (e.g., spouse, kids, friends)

Nighttime REFLECTION

- ∞ WIN: I am _Celebrating_ myself for _____
- ∞ CHALLENGE: It felt hard when _____
  - ♥ I choose to see this as an opportunity to _____
  - ♥ Say aloud: *I forgive, and I release this challenge with love. *Inhale, Exhale**
- ∞ SUPPORT: I felt supported today by/when _____
  _____
- ∞ GRATITUDE: I am grateful for _____
  _____
- ∞ INTENTION: My intention for the morning is _____

Tuesday

Morning PEP TALK

- ∞ In the mirror, with one hand on your heart: I LOVE YOU. YOU'VE GOT THIS, _____!

(NAME)
- ∞ Affirmation: I (AM) _____
- ∞ I am grateful for (3+) _____
  _____
- ∞ I thank my body for _____
- ∞ HABIT TRACKER, Day ___ of 30

Wellbeing ACTIONS

- ☐ Today, I GET to _____ for me (prompts: JOY-FULL List p.15)
- ☐ Today, I GET to _____ my baby.
- ☐ Today, I GET to _____ for/with _____

(e.g., spouse, kids, friends)

Nighttime REFLECTION

- ∞ WIN: I am *Celebrating* myself for _____
- ∞ CHALLENGE: It felt hard when _____
  - ♥ I choose to see this as an opportunity to _____
  - ♥ Say aloud: *I forgive, and I release this challenge with love. *Inhale, Exhale**
- ∞ SUPPORT: I felt supported today by/when _____
  _____
- ∞ GRATITUDE: I am grateful for _____
  _____
- ∞ INTENTION: My intention for the morning is _____

Wednesday

Morning PEP TALK

- ∞ In the mirror, with one hand on your heart: I LOVE YOU. YOU'VE GOT THIS, _____!
  (NAME)
- ∞ Affirmation: I (AM) _____
- ∞ I am grateful for (3+) _____
  _____
- ∞ I thank my body for _____
- ∞ HABIT TRACKER, Day ___ of 30

Wellbeing ACTIONS

- ☐ Today, I GET to _____ for me (prompts: JOY-FULL List p.15)
- ☐ Today, I GET to _____ my baby.
- ☐ Today, I GET to _____ for/with _____
  (e.g., spouse, kids, friends)

Nighttime REFLECTION

- ∞ WIN: I am _Celebrating_ myself for _____
- ∞ CHALLENGE: It felt hard when _____
  - ♥ I choose to see this as an opportunity to _____
  - ♥ Say aloud: *I forgive, and I release this challenge with love.*
    Inhale, Exhale
- ∞ SUPPORT: I felt supported today by/when _____
  _____
- ∞ GRATITUDE: I am grateful for _____
  _____
- ∞ INTENTION: My intention for the morning is _____

Thursday

Morning PEP TALK

- ∞ In the mirror, with one hand on your heart: I LOVE YOU. YOU'VE GOT THIS, _____!
  (NAME)
- ∞ Affirmation: I (AM) _____
- ∞ I am grateful for (3+) _____
  _____
- ∞ I thank my body for _____
- ∞ HABIT TRACKER, Day ___ of 30

Wellbeing ACTIONS

- ☐ Today, I GET to _____ for me (prompts: JOY-FULL List p.15)
- ☐ Today, I GET to _____ my baby.
- ☐ Today, I GET to _____ for/with _____
  (e.g., spouse, kids, friends)

Nighttime REFLECTION

- ∞ WIN: I am *Celebrating* myself for _____
- ∞ CHALLENGE: It felt hard when _____
  - ♥ I choose to see this as an opportunity to _____
  - ♥ Say aloud: *I forgive, and I release this challenge with love. *Inhale, Exhale**
- ∞ SUPPORT: I felt supported today by/when _____
  _____
- ∞ GRATITUDE: I am grateful for _____
  _____
- ∞ INTENTION: My intention for the morning is _____

Friday

Morning PEP TALK

- ∞ In the mirror, with one hand on your heart: I LOVE YOU. YOU'VE GOT THIS, _____!
  (NAME)
- ∞ Affirmation: I (AM) _____
- ∞ I am grateful for (3+) _____
  _____
- ∞ I thank my body for _____
- ∞ HABIT TRACKER, Day ___ of 30

Wellbeing ACTIONS

- ☐ Today, I GET to _____ for me (prompts: JOY-FULL List p.15)
- ☐ Today, I GET to _____ my baby.
- ☐ Today, I GET to _____ for/with _____
  (e.g., spouse, kids, friends)

Nighttime REFLECTION

- ∞ WIN: I am _Celebrating_ myself for _____
- ∞ CHALLENGE: It felt hard when _____
  - ♥ I choose to see this as an opportunity to _____
  - ♥ Say aloud: *I forgive, and I release this challenge with love.* *Inhale, Exhale*
- ∞ SUPPORT: I felt supported today by/when _____
  _____
- ∞ GRATITUDE: I am grateful for _____
  _____
- ∞ INTENTION: My intention for the morning is _____

Saturday

Morning PEP TALK

- ∞ In the mirror, with one hand on your heart: I LOVE YOU. YOU'VE GOT THIS, _____!
  (NAME)
- ∞ Affirmation: I (AM) _____
- ∞ I am grateful for (3+) _____
  _____
- ∞ I thank my body for _____
- ∞ HABIT TRACKER, Day ___ of 30

Wellbeing ACTIONS

- ☐ Today, I GET to _____ for me (prompts: JOY-FULL List p.15)
- ☐ Today, I GET to _____ my baby.
- ☐ Today, I GET to _____ for/with _____
  (e.g., spouse, kids, friends)

Nighttime REFLECTION

- ∞ WIN: I am *Celebrating* myself for _____
- ∞ CHALLENGE: It felt hard when _____
  - ♥ I choose to see this as an opportunity to _____
  - ♥ Say aloud: *I forgive, and I release this challenge with love. *Inhale, Exhale**
- ∞ SUPPORT: I felt supported today by/when _____
  _____
- ∞ GRATITUDE: I am grateful for _____
  _____
- ∞ INTENTION: My intention for the morning is _____

Sunday

Morning PEP TALK

- ∞ In the mirror, with one hand on your heart: I LOVE YOU. YOU'VE GOT THIS, _____!
  (NAME)
- ∞ Affirmation: I (AM) _____
- ∞ I am grateful for (3+) _____
  _____
- ∞ I thank my body for _____
- ∞ HABIT TRACKER, Day ___ of 30

Wellbeing ACTIONS

- ☐ Today, I GET to _____ for me (prompts: JOY-FULL List p.15)
- ☐ Today, I GET to _____ my baby.
- ☐ Today, I GET to _____ for/with _____
  (e.g., spouse, kids, friends)

Nighttime REFLECTION

- ∞ WIN: I am *Celebrating* myself for _____
- ∞ CHALLENGE: It felt hard when _____
  - ♥ I choose to see this as an opportunity to _____
  - ♥ Say aloud: *I forgive, and I release this challenge with love. *Inhale, Exhale**
- ∞ SUPPORT: I felt supported today by/when _____
  _____
- ∞ GRATITUDE: I am grateful for _____
  _____
- ∞ INTENTION: My intention for the morning is _____

What's happening this week

Week of: _____

- ♥ Affirmation: I _____

- ♥ I will show myself grace this week by _____

- ♥ I am looking forward to _____

- ♥ I get to ask for support with _____

   By (action step) _____

☐ Review #2-6 from the Monthly Wellbeing Check-in. Take a moment to visualize yourself integrating these feelings, actions, and thoughts now, as well as throughout this week.

☐ Review upcoming appointments and set an alarm in your phone as needed.

Grocery list:
(TIP: Record here and take a picture to bring ease to the next grocery store trip.)

_____	_____	_____
_____	_____	_____
_____	_____	_____
_____	_____	_____
_____	_____	_____
_____	_____	_____
_____	_____	_____

Monday

Morning PEP TALK

- ∞ In the mirror, with one hand on your heart: I LOVE YOU. YOU'VE GOT THIS, _____!
  (NAME)
- ∞ Affirmation: I (AM) _____
- ∞ I am grateful for (3+) _____
  _____
- ∞ I thank my body for _____
- ∞ HABIT TRACKER, Day ___ of 30

Wellbeing ACTIONS

- ☐ Today, I GET to _____ for me (prompts: JOY-FULL List p.15)
- ☐ Today, I GET to _____ my baby.
- ☐ Today, I GET to _____ for/with _____
  (e.g., spouse, kids, friends)

Nighttime REFLECTION

- ∞ WIN: I am *Celebrating* myself for _____
- ∞ CHALLENGE: It felt hard when _____
  - ♥ I choose to see this as an opportunity to _____
  - ♥ Say aloud: *I forgive, and I release this challenge with love. *Inhale, Exhale**
- ∞ SUPPORT: I felt supported today by/when _____
  _____
- ∞ GRATITUDE: I am grateful for _____
  _____
- ∞ INTENTION: My intention for the morning is _____

Tuesday

Morning PEP TALK

- ∞ In the mirror, with one hand on your heart: I LOVE YOU. YOU'VE GOT THIS, _____ !
  (NAME)
- ∞ Affirmation: I (AM) _____
- ∞ I am grateful for (3+) _____
  _____
- ∞ I thank my body for _____
- ∞ HABIT TRACKER, Day ___ of 30

Wellbeing ACTIONS

- ☐ Today, I GET to _____ for me (prompts: JOY-FULL List p.15)
- ☐ Today, I GET to _____ my baby.
- ☐ Today, I GET to _____ for/with _____
  (e.g., spouse, kids, friends)

Nighttime REFLECTION

- ∞ WIN: I am _Celebrating_ myself for _____
- ∞ CHALLENGE: It felt hard when _____
  - ♥ I choose to see this as an opportunity to _____
  - ♥ Say aloud: *I forgive, and I release this challenge with love.* *Inhale, Exhale*
- ∞ SUPPORT: I felt supported today by/when _____
  _____
- ∞ GRATITUDE: I am grateful for _____
  _____
- ∞ INTENTION: My intention for the morning is _____

Wednesday

Morning PEP TALK

- ∞ In the mirror, with one hand on your heart: I LOVE YOU. YOU'VE GOT THIS, _____!
  (NAME)
- ∞ Affirmation: I (AM) _____
- ∞ I am grateful for (3+) _____
  _____
- ∞ I thank my body for _____
- ∞ HABIT TRACKER, Day ___ of 30

Wellbeing ACTIONS

- ☐ Today, I GET to _____ for me (prompts: JOY-FULL List p.15)
- ☐ Today, I GET to _____ my baby.
- ☐ Today, I GET to _____ for/with _____
  (e.g., spouse, kids, friends)

Nighttime REFLECTION

- ∞ WIN: I am _Celebrating_ myself for _____
- ∞ CHALLENGE: It felt hard when _____
  - ♥ I choose to see this as an opportunity to _____
  - ♥ Say aloud: *I forgive, and I release this challenge with love.*
    Inhale, Exhale
- ∞ SUPPORT: I felt supported today by/when _____
  _____
- ∞ GRATITUDE: I am grateful for _____
  _____
- ∞ INTENTION: My intention for the morning is _____

Thursday

Morning PEP TALK

- ∞ In the mirror, with one hand on your heart: I LOVE YOU. YOU'VE GOT THIS, _____!
  (NAME)
- ∞ Affirmation: I (AM) _____
- ∞ I am grateful for (3+) _____
  _____
- ∞ I thank my body for _____
- ∞ HABIT TRACKER, Day ___ of 30

Wellbeing ACTIONS

- ☐ Today, I GET to _____ for me (prompts: JOY-FULL List p.15)
- ☐ Today, I GET to _____ my baby.
- ☐ Today, I GET to _____ for/with _____
  (e.g., spouse, kids, friends)

Nighttime REFLECTION

- ∞ WIN: I am *Celebrating* myself for _____
- ∞ CHALLENGE: It felt hard when _____
  - ♥ I choose to see this as an opportunity to _____
  - ♥ Say aloud: *I forgive, and I release this challenge with love.* *Inhale, Exhale*
- ∞ SUPPORT: I felt supported today by/when _____
  _____
- ∞ GRATITUDE: I am grateful for _____
  _____
- ∞ INTENTION: My intention for the morning is _____

Friday

Morning PEP TALK

- ∞ In the mirror, with one hand on your heart: I LOVE YOU. YOU'VE GOT THIS, _____!
(NAME)
- ∞ Affirmation: I (AM) _____
- ∞ I am grateful for (3+) _____
_____
- ∞ I thank my body for _____
- ∞ HABIT TRACKER, Day ___ of 30

Wellbeing ACTIONS

- ☐ Today, I GET to _____ for me (prompts: JOY-FULL List p.15)
- ☐ Today, I GET to _____ my baby.
- ☐ Today, I GET to _____ for/with _____
(e.g., spouse, kids, friends)

Nighttime REFLECTION

- ∞ WIN: I am *Celebrating* myself for _____
- ∞ CHALLENGE: It felt hard when _____
  - ♥ I choose to see this as an opportunity to _____
  - ♥ Say aloud: *I forgive, and I release this challenge with love. *Inhale, Exhale**
- ∞ SUPPORT: I felt supported today by/when _____
_____
- ∞ GRATITUDE: I am grateful for _____
_____
- ∞ INTENTION: My intention for the morning is _____

Saturday

Morning PEP TALK

- ∞ In the mirror, with one hand on your heart: I LOVE YOU. YOU'VE GOT THIS, _____!
  (NAME)
- ∞ Affirmation: I (AM) _____
- ∞ I am grateful for (3+) _____
  _____
- ∞ I thank my body for _____
- ∞ HABIT TRACKER, Day ___ of 30

Wellbeing ACTIONS

- ☐ Today, I GET to _____ for me (prompts: JOY-FULL List p.15)
- ☐ Today, I GET to _____ my baby.
- ☐ Today, I GET to _____ for/with _____
  (e.g., spouse, kids, friends)

Nighttime REFLECTION

- ∞ WIN: I am *Celebrating* myself for _____
- ∞ CHALLENGE: It felt hard when _____
  - ♥ I choose to see this as an opportunity to _____
  - ♥ Say aloud: *I forgive, and I release this challenge with love. *Inhale, Exhale**
- ∞ SUPPORT: I felt supported today by/when _____
  _____
- ∞ GRATITUDE: I am grateful for _____
  _____
- ∞ INTENTION: My intention for the morning is _____

Sunday

Morning PEP TALK

- ∞ In the mirror, with one hand on your heart: I LOVE YOU. YOU'VE GOT THIS, _____!
  (NAME)
- ∞ Affirmation: I (AM) _____
- ∞ I am grateful for (3+) _____
  _____
- ∞ I thank my body for _____
- ∞ HABIT TRACKER, Day ___ of 30

Wellbeing ACTIONS

- ☐ Today, I GET to _____ for me (prompts: JOY-FULL List p.15)
- ☐ Today, I GET to _____ my baby.
- ☐ Today, I GET to _____ for/with _____
  (e.g., spouse, kids, friends)

Nighttime REFLECTION

- ∞ WIN: I am *Celebrating* myself for _____
- ∞ CHALLENGE: It felt hard when _____
  - ♥ I choose to see this as an opportunity to _____
  - ♥ Say aloud: *I forgive, and I release this challenge with love. *Inhale, Exhale**
- ∞ SUPPORT: I felt supported today by/when _____
  _____
- ∞ GRATITUDE: I am grateful for _____
  _____
- ∞ INTENTION: My intention for the morning is _____

What's happening this week

Week of: _____

- ♥ Affirmation: I _____

- ♥ I will show myself grace this week by _____

- ♥ I am looking forward to _____

- ♥ I get to ask for support with _____

    By (action step) _____

- ☐ Review #2-6 from the Monthly Wellbeing Check-in. Take a moment to visualize yourself integrating these feelings, actions, and thoughts now, as well as throughout this week.

- ☐ Review upcoming appointments and set an alarm in your phone as needed.

Grocery list:
(TIP: Record here and take a picture to bring ease to the next grocery store trip.)

_____	_____	_____
_____	_____	_____
_____	_____	_____
_____	_____	_____
_____	_____	_____
_____	_____	_____
_____	_____	_____

Monday

Morning PEP TALK

- ∞ In the mirror, with one hand on your heart: I LOVE YOU. YOU'VE GOT THIS, _____!
  (NAME)
- ∞ Affirmation: I (AM) _____
- ∞ I am grateful for (3+) _____
  _____
- ∞ I thank my body for _____
- ∞ HABIT TRACKER, Day ___ of 30

Wellbeing ACTIONS

- ☐ Today, I GET to _____ for me (prompts: JOY-FULL List p.15)
- ☐ Today, I GET to _____ my baby.
- ☐ Today, I GET to _____ for/with _____
  (e.g., spouse, kids, friends)

Nighttime REFLECTION

- ∞ WIN: I am *Celebrating* myself for _____
- ∞ CHALLENGE: It felt hard when _____
  - ♥ I choose to see this as an opportunity to _____
  - ♥ Say aloud: *I forgive, and I release this challenge with love. *Inhale, Exhale**
- ∞ SUPPORT: I felt supported today by/when _____
  _____
- ∞ GRATITUDE: I am grateful for _____
  _____
- ∞ INTENTION: My intention for the morning is _____

Tuesday

Morning PEP TALK

- ∞ In the mirror, with one hand on your heart: I LOVE YOU. YOU'VE GOT THIS, _____!
  (NAME)
- ∞ Affirmation: I (AM) _____
- ∞ I am grateful for (3+) _____
  _____
- ∞ I thank my body for _____
- ∞ HABIT TRACKER, Day ___ of 30

Wellbeing ACTIONS

- ☐ Today, I GET to _____ for me (prompts: JOY-FULL List p.15)
- ☐ Today, I GET to _____ my baby.
- ☐ Today, I GET to _____ for/with _____
  (e.g., spouse, kids, friends)

Nighttime REFLECTION

- ∞ WIN: I am _Celebrating_ myself for _____
- ∞ CHALLENGE: It felt hard when _____
  - ♥ I choose to see this as an opportunity to _____
  - ♥ Say aloud: *I forgive, and I release this challenge with love. *Inhale, Exhale**
- ∞ SUPPORT: I felt supported today by/when _____
  _____
- ∞ GRATITUDE: I am grateful for _____
  _____
- ∞ INTENTION: My intention for the morning is _____

Wednesday

Morning PEP TALK

- ∞ In the mirror, with one hand on your heart: I LOVE YOU. YOU'VE GOT THIS, _____!
  (NAME)
- ∞ Affirmation: I (AM) _____
- ∞ I am grateful for (3+) _____
  _____
- ∞ I thank my body for _____
- ∞ HABIT TRACKER, Day ___ of 30

Wellbeing ACTIONS

- ☐ Today, I GET to _____ for me (prompts: JOY-FULL List p.15)
- ☐ Today, I GET to _____ my baby.
- ☐ Today, I GET to _____ for/with _____
  (e.g., spouse, kids, friends)

Nighttime REFLECTION

- ∞ WIN: I am <u>Celebrating</u> myself for _____
- ∞ CHALLENGE: It felt hard when _____
  - ♥ I choose to see this as an opportunity to _____
  - ♥ Say aloud: *I forgive, and I release this challenge with love.*
    Inhale, Exhale
- ∞ SUPPORT: I felt supported today by/when _____
  _____
- ∞ GRATITUDE: I am grateful for _____
  _____
- ∞ INTENTION: My intention for the morning is _____

Thursday

Morning PEP TALK

- ∞ In the mirror, with one hand on your heart: I LOVE YOU. YOU'VE GOT THIS, _____!
  (NAME)
- ∞ Affirmation: I (AM) _____
- ∞ I am grateful for (3+) _____
  _____
- ∞ I thank my body for _____
- ∞ HABIT TRACKER, Day ___ of 30

Wellbeing ACTIONS

- ☐ Today, I GET to _____ for me (prompts: JOY-FULL List p.15)
- ☐ Today, I GET to _____ my baby.
- ☐ Today, I GET to _____ for/with _____
  (e.g., spouse, kids, friends)

Nighttime REFLECTION

- ∞ WIN: I am <u>Celebrating</u> myself for _____
- ∞ CHALLENGE: It felt hard when _____
    - ♥ I choose to see this as an opportunity to _____
    - ♥ Say aloud: *I forgive, and I release this challenge with love. *Inhale, Exhale**
- ∞ SUPPORT: I felt supported today by/when _____
  _____
- ∞ GRATITUDE: I am grateful for _____
  _____
- ∞ INTENTION: My intention for the morning is _____

Friday

Morning PEP TALK

- ∞ In the mirror, with one hand on your heart: I LOVE YOU. YOU'VE GOT THIS, _____!
  (NAME)
- ∞ Affirmation: I (AM) _____
- ∞ I am grateful for (3+) _____
  _____
- ∞ I thank my body for _____
- ∞ HABIT TRACKER, Day ___ of 30

Wellbeing ACTIONS

- ☐ Today, I GET to _____ for me (prompts: JOY-FULL List p.15)
- ☐ Today, I GET to _____ my baby.
- ☐ Today, I GET to _____ for/with _____
  (e.g., spouse, kids, friends)

Nighttime REFLECTION

- ∞ WIN: I am *Celebrating* myself for _____
- ∞ CHALLENGE: It felt hard when _____
  - ♥ I choose to see this as an opportunity to _____
  - ♥ Say aloud: *I forgive, and I release this challenge with love. *Inhale, Exhale**
- ∞ SUPPORT: I felt supported today by/when _____
  _____
- ∞ GRATITUDE: I am grateful for _____
  _____
- ∞ INTENTION: My intention for the morning is _____

Saturday

Morning PEP TALK

- ∞ In the mirror, with one hand on your heart: I LOVE YOU. YOU'VE GOT THIS, _____ !
  (NAME)
- ∞ Affirmation: I (AM) _____
- ∞ I am grateful for (3+) _____
  _____
- ∞ I thank my body for _____
- ∞ HABIT TRACKER, Day ___ of 30

Wellbeing ACTIONS

- ☐ Today, I GET to _____ for me (prompts: JOY-FULL List p.15)
- ☐ Today, I GET to _____ my baby.
- ☐ Today, I GET to _____ for/with _____
  (e.g., spouse, kids, friends)

Nighttime REFLECTION

- ∞ WIN: I am _Celebrating_ myself for _____
- ∞ CHALLENGE: It felt hard when _____
  - ♥ I choose to see this as an opportunity to _____
  - ♥ Say aloud: *I forgive, and I release this challenge with love. *Inhale, Exhale**
- ∞ SUPPORT: I felt supported today by/when _____
  _____
- ∞ GRATITUDE: I am grateful for _____
  _____
- ∞ INTENTION: My intention for the morning is _____

Sunday

Morning PEP TALK

- ∞ In the mirror, with one hand on your heart: I LOVE YOU. YOU'VE GOT THIS, _____!
  (NAME)
- ∞ Affirmation: I (AM) _____
- ∞ I am grateful for (3+) _____
  _____
- ∞ I thank my body for _____
- ∞ HABIT TRACKER, Day ___ of 30

Wellbeing ACTIONS

- ☐ Today, I GET to _____ for me (prompts: JOY-FULL List p.15)
- ☐ Today, I GET to _____ my baby.
- ☐ Today, I GET to _____ for/with _____
  (e.g., spouse, kids, friends)

Nighttime REFLECTION

- ∞ WIN: I am _Celebrating_ myself for _____
- ∞ CHALLENGE: It felt hard when _____
  - ♥ I choose to see this as an opportunity to _____
  - ♥ Say aloud: *I forgive, and I release this challenge with love.* *Inhale, Exhale*
- ∞ SUPPORT: I felt supported today by/when _____
  _____
- ∞ GRATITUDE: I am grateful for _____
  _____
- ∞ INTENTION: My intention for the morning is _____

Monthly Recap

- ♥ I am Celebrating _____!
    - ◊ In my head, I feel _____
    - ◊ In my heart, I feel _____
    - ◊ In my body, I feel _____
- ♥ My favourite activities this month were _____
  _____
    because _____
- ♥ My favourite affirmations this month were _____
  _____
    because _____
- ♥ It felt hard when _____
    From this, I learned _____
- ♥ I feel more joy and ease in my life when I _____
  _____
- ♥ I felt most supported this month when _____
- ♥ I am grateful for _____
- ♥ The boundary I set up at the beginning of the month helped me by
  _____
- ♥ I am celebrating my new habit this month!
    I am bringing this new habit with me into next month because (impact)
  _____
- ♥ Special milestones/memories (date and event):

MONTH:

Free write/Notes/Lessons/Draw

MONTH: _____

SUNDAY	MONDAY	TUESDAY	WEDNESDAY
___	___	___	___
___	___	___	___
___	___	___	___
___	___	___	___
___	___	___	___

Record special dates, appointments, milestones, etc.

THURSDAY	FRIDAY	SATURDAY	NOTES
___	___	___	
___	___	___	
___	___	___	
___	___	___	
___	___	___	

Monthly Wellbeing Check-in

MONTH: _____

1. How do I feel right now?

    ◊ In my head (mentally): _____
    _____

    ◊ In my heart (emotionally): _____
    _____

    ◊ In my body (physically): _____
    _____

2. How do I desire to feel?

    ◊ In my head (mentally): _____
    _____

    ◊ In my heart (emotionally): _____
    _____

    ◊ In my body (physically): _____
    _____

3. What actions can I take to help me feel the way I described above? What thoughts can I have to help me feel this way?

    ◊ In my head (mentally): _____
    _____

    ◊ In my heart (emotionally): _____
    _____

    ◊ In my body (physically): _____
    _____

4. What am I excited for this month? _____

_____

5. What boundary am I setting up this month? _____

_____

- ◊ Action(s) to set up this boundary: _____

    _____

6. HABIT TRACKER (e.g., action/thought you wrote about for your desired feeling in #3):

I _____ am developing the habit of _____ this month.
  (NAME)

Picture this as a habit already. How do I feel? How am I showing up? What is different?

_____

_____

_____

_____

_____

_____

I understand that I may miss a day. I will show myself grace and re-commit the next day.

This habit supports me.

I am doing my best and I am Thriving!

What's happening this week

Week of: _____

- ♥ Affirmation: I _____

- ♥ I will show myself grace this week by _____

- ♥ I am looking forward to _____

- ♥ I get to ask for support with _____

    By (action step) _____

- ☐ Review #2-6 from the Monthly Wellbeing Check-in. Take a moment to visualize yourself integrating these feelings, actions, and thoughts now, as well as throughout this week.

- ☐ Review upcoming appointments and set an alarm in your phone as needed.

Grocery list:
(TIP: Record here and take a picture to bring ease to the next grocery store trip.)

_____	_____	_____
_____	_____	_____
_____	_____	_____
_____	_____	_____
_____	_____	_____
_____	_____	_____
_____	_____	_____

Monday

Morning PEP TALK

- ∞ In the mirror, with one hand on your heart: I LOVE YOU. YOU'VE GOT THIS, _____!
  (NAME)
- ∞ Affirmation: I (AM) _____
- ∞ I am grateful for (3+) _____
  _____
- ∞ I thank my body for _____
- ∞ HABIT TRACKER, Day ___ of 30

Wellbeing ACTIONS

- ☐ Today, I GET to _____ for me (prompts: JOY-FULL List p.15)
- ☐ Today, I GET to _____ my baby.
- ☐ Today, I GET to _____ for/with _____
  (e.g., spouse, kids, friends)

Nighttime REFLECTION

- ∞ WIN: I am <u>Celebrating</u> myself for _____
- ∞ CHALLENGE: It felt hard when _____
  - ♥ I choose to see this as an opportunity to _____
  - ♥ Say aloud: *I forgive, and I release this challenge with love.*
    Inhale, Exhale
- ∞ SUPPORT: I felt supported today by/when _____
  _____
- ∞ GRATITUDE: I am grateful for _____
  _____
- ∞ INTENTION: My intention for the morning is _____

Tuesday

Morning PEP TALK

- ∞ In the mirror, with one hand on your heart: I LOVE YOU. YOU'VE GOT THIS, _____!
  (NAME)
- ∞ Affirmation: I (AM) _____
- ∞ I am grateful for (3+) _____
  _____
- ∞ I thank my body for _____
- ∞ HABIT TRACKER, Day ___ of 30

Wellbeing ACTIONS

- ☐ Today, I GET to _____ for me (prompts: JOY-FULL List p.15)
- ☐ Today, I GET to _____ my baby.
- ☐ Today, I GET to _____ for/with _____
  (e.g., spouse, kids, friends)

Nighttime REFLECTION

- ∞ WIN: I am *Celebrating* myself for _____
- ∞ CHALLENGE: It felt hard when _____
  - ♥ I choose to see this as an opportunity to _____
  - ♥ Say aloud: *I forgive, and I release this challenge with love. *Inhale, Exhale**
- ∞ SUPPORT: I felt supported today by/when _____
  _____
- ∞ GRATITUDE: I am grateful for _____
  _____
- ∞ INTENTION: My intention for the morning is _____

Wednesday

Morning PEP TALK

- ∞ In the mirror, with one hand on your heart: I LOVE YOU. YOU'VE GOT THIS, _____!
  (NAME)
- ∞ Affirmation: I (AM) _____
- ∞ I am grateful for (3+) _____
  _____
- ∞ I thank my body for _____
- ∞ HABIT TRACKER, Day ___ of 30

Wellbeing ACTIONS

- ☐ Today, I GET to _____ for me (prompts: JOY-FULL List p.15)
- ☐ Today, I GET to _____ my baby.
- ☐ Today, I GET to _____ for/with _____
  (e.g., spouse, kids, friends)

Nighttime REFLECTION

- ∞ WIN: I am _Celebrating_ myself for _____
- ∞ CHALLENGE: It felt hard when _____
    - ♥ I choose to see this as an opportunity to _____
    - ♥ Say aloud: *I forgive, and I release this challenge with love.*
      Inhale, Exhale
- ∞ SUPPORT: I felt supported today by/when _____
  _____
- ∞ GRATITUDE: I am grateful for _____
  _____
- ∞ INTENTION: My intention for the morning is _____

Thursday

Morning PEP TALK

- ∞ In the mirror, with one hand on your heart: I LOVE YOU. YOU'VE GOT THIS, _____!

(NAME)
- ∞ Affirmation: I (AM) _____
- ∞ I am grateful for (3+) _____
  _____
- ∞ I thank my body for _____
- ∞ HABIT TRACKER, Day ___ of 30

Wellbeing ACTIONS

- ☐ Today, I GET to _____ for me (prompts: JOY-FULL List p.15)
- ☐ Today, I GET to _____ my baby.
- ☐ Today, I GET to _____ for/with _____

(e.g., spouse, kids, friends)

Nighttime REFLECTION

- ∞ WIN: I am *Celebrating* myself for _____
- ∞ CHALLENGE: It felt hard when _____
    - ♥ I choose to see this as an opportunity to _____
    - ♥ Say aloud: *I forgive, and I release this challenge with love. *Inhale, Exhale**
- ∞ SUPPORT: I felt supported today by/when _____
  _____
- ∞ GRATITUDE: I am grateful for _____
  _____
- ∞ INTENTION: My intention for the morning is _____

Friday

Morning PEP TALK

- ∞ In the mirror, with one hand on your heart: I LOVE YOU. YOU'VE GOT THIS, _____!
  (NAME)
- ∞ Affirmation: I (AM) _____
- ∞ I am grateful for (3+) _____
  _____
- ∞ I thank my body for _____
- ∞ HABIT TRACKER, Day ___ of 30

Wellbeing ACTIONS

- ☐ Today, I GET to _____ for me (prompts: JOY-FULL List p.15)
- ☐ Today, I GET to _____ my baby.
- ☐ Today, I GET to _____ for/with _____
  (e.g., spouse, kids, friends)

Nighttime REFLECTION

- ∞ WIN: I am *Celebrating* myself for _____
- ∞ CHALLENGE: It felt hard when _____
  - ♥ I choose to see this as an opportunity to _____
  - ♥ Say aloud: *I forgive, and I release this challenge with love. *Inhale, Exhale**
- ∞ SUPPORT: I felt supported today by/when _____
  _____
- ∞ GRATITUDE: I am grateful for _____
  _____
- ∞ INTENTION: My intention for the morning is _____

Saturday

Morning PEP TALK

- ∞ In the mirror, with one hand on your heart: I LOVE YOU. YOU'VE GOT THIS, _____!
  (NAME)
- ∞ Affirmation: I (AM) _____
- ∞ I am grateful for (3+) _____
  _____
- ∞ I thank my body for _____
- ∞ HABIT TRACKER, Day ___ of 30

Wellbeing ACTIONS

- ☐ Today, I GET to _____ for me (prompts: JOY-FULL List p.15)
- ☐ Today, I GET to _____ my baby.
- ☐ Today, I GET to _____ for/with _____
  (e.g., spouse, kids, friends)

Nighttime REFLECTION

- ∞ WIN: I am *Celebrating* myself for _____
- ∞ CHALLENGE: It felt hard when _____
  - ♥ I choose to see this as an opportunity to _____
  - ♥ Say aloud: *I forgive, and I release this challenge with love. *Inhale, Exhale**
- ∞ SUPPORT: I felt supported today by/when _____
  _____
- ∞ GRATITUDE: I am grateful for _____
  _____
- ∞ INTENTION: My intention for the morning is _____

Sunday

Morning PEP TALK

- ∞ In the mirror, with one hand on your heart: I LOVE YOU. YOU'VE GOT THIS, _____!
  (NAME)
- ∞ Affirmation: I (AM) _____
- ∞ I am grateful for (3+) _____
  _____
- ∞ I thank my body for _____
- ∞ HABIT TRACKER, Day ___ of 30

Wellbeing ACTIONS

- ☐ Today, I GET to _____ for me (prompts: JOY-FULL List p.15)
- ☐ Today, I GET to _____ my baby.
- ☐ Today, I GET to _____ for/with _____
  (e.g., spouse, kids, friends)

Nighttime REFLECTION

- ∞ WIN: I am *Celebrating* myself for _____
- ∞ CHALLENGE: It felt hard when _____
  - ♥ I choose to see this as an opportunity to _____
  - ♥ Say aloud: *I forgive, and I release this challenge with love. *Inhale, Exhale**
- ∞ SUPPORT: I felt supported today by/when _____
  _____
- ∞ GRATITUDE: I am grateful for _____
  _____
- ∞ INTENTION: My intention for the morning is _____

What's happening this week

Week of: _____

- ♥ Affirmation: I _____

- ♥ I will show myself grace this week by _____

- ♥ I am looking forward to _____

- ♥ I get to ask for support with _____

    By (action step) _____

- ☐ Review #2-6 from the Monthly Wellbeing Check-in. Take a moment to visualize yourself integrating these feelings, actions, and thoughts now, as well as throughout this week.

- ☐ Review upcoming appointments and set an alarm in your phone as needed.

Grocery list:
(TIP: Record here and take a picture to bring ease to the next grocery store trip.)

_____	_____	_____
_____	_____	_____
_____	_____	_____
_____	_____	_____
_____	_____	_____
_____	_____	_____
_____	_____	_____

Monday

Morning PEP TALK

- ∞ In the mirror, with one hand on your heart: I LOVE YOU. YOU'VE GOT THIS, _____!
  (NAME)
- ∞ Affirmation: I (AM) _____
- ∞ I am grateful for (3+) _____
  _____
- ∞ I thank my body for _____
- ∞ HABIT TRACKER, Day ___ of 30

Wellbeing ACTIONS

- ☐ Today, I GET to _____ for me (prompts: JOY-FULL List p.15)
- ☐ Today, I GET to _____ my baby.
- ☐ Today, I GET to _____ for/with _____
  (e.g., spouse, kids, friends)

Nighttime REFLECTION

- ∞ WIN: I am *Celebrating* myself for _____
- ∞ CHALLENGE: It felt hard when _____
  - ♥ I choose to see this as an opportunity to _____
  - ♥ Say aloud: *I forgive, and I release this challenge with love. *Inhale, Exhale**
- ∞ SUPPORT: I felt supported today by/when _____
  _____
- ∞ GRATITUDE: I am grateful for _____
  _____
- ∞ INTENTION: My intention for the morning is _____

Tuesday

Morning PEP TALK

- ∞ In the mirror, with one hand on your heart: I LOVE YOU. YOU'VE GOT THIS, _____!
  (NAME)
- ∞ Affirmation: I (AM) _____
- ∞ I am grateful for (3+) _____
  _____
- ∞ I thank my body for _____
- ∞ HABIT TRACKER, Day ___ of 30

Wellbeing ACTIONS

- ☐ Today, I GET to _____ for me (prompts: JOY-FULL List p.15)
- ☐ Today, I GET to _____ my baby.
- ☐ Today, I GET to _____ for/with _____
  (e.g., spouse, kids, friends)

Nighttime REFLECTION

- ∞ WIN: I am _Celebrating_ myself for _____
- ∞ CHALLENGE: It felt hard when _____
  - ♥ I choose to see this as an opportunity to _____
  - ♥ Say aloud: *I forgive, and I release this challenge with love. *Inhale, Exhale**
- ∞ SUPPORT: I felt supported today by/when _____
  _____
- ∞ GRATITUDE: I am grateful for _____
  _____
- ∞ INTENTION: My intention for the morning is _____

Wednesday

Morning PEP TALK

- ∞ In the mirror, with one hand on your heart: I LOVE YOU. YOU'VE GOT THIS, _____!
  (NAME)
- ∞ Affirmation: I (AM) _____
- ∞ I am grateful for (3+) _____
  _____
- ∞ I thank my body for _____
- ∞ HABIT TRACKER, Day ___ of 30

Wellbeing ACTIONS

- ☐ Today, I GET to _____ for me (prompts: JOY-FULL List p.15)
- ☐ Today, I GET to _____ my baby.
- ☐ Today, I GET to _____ for/with _____
  (e.g., spouse, kids, friends)

Nighttime REFLECTION

- ∞ WIN: I am *Celebrating* myself for _____
- ∞ CHALLENGE: It felt hard when _____
  - ♥ I choose to see this as an opportunity to _____
  - ♥ Say aloud: *I forgive, and I release this challenge with love. *Inhale, Exhale**
- ∞ SUPPORT: I felt supported today by/when _____
  _____
- ∞ GRATITUDE: I am grateful for _____
  _____
- ∞ INTENTION: My intention for the morning is _____

<u>Thursday</u>

Morning PEP TALK

- ∞ In the mirror, with one hand on your heart: I LOVE YOU. YOU'VE GOT THIS, _____ !
  (NAME)
- ∞ Affirmation: I (AM) _____
- ∞ I am grateful for (3+) _____

  _____

- ∞ I thank my body for _____
- ∞ HABIT TRACKER, Day ___ of 30

Wellbeing ACTIONS

- ☐ Today, I GET to _____ for me (prompts: JOY-FULL List p.15)
- ☐ Today, I GET to _____ my baby.
- ☐ Today, I GET to _____ for/with _____
  (e.g., spouse, kids, friends)

Nighttime REFLECTION

- ∞ WIN: I am *Celebrating* myself for _____
- ∞ CHALLENGE: It felt hard when _____
    - ♥ I choose to see this as an opportunity to _____
    - ♥ Say aloud: *I forgive, and I release this challenge with love. *Inhale, Exhale**
- ∞ SUPPORT: I felt supported today by/when _____

  _____

- ∞ GRATITUDE: I am grateful for _____

  _____

- ∞ INTENTION: My intention for the morning is _____

Friday

Morning PEP TALK

- ∞ In the mirror, with one hand on your heart: I LOVE YOU. YOU'VE GOT THIS, _____!
  (NAME)
- ∞ Affirmation: I (AM) _____
- ∞ I am grateful for (3+) _____
  _____
- ∞ I thank my body for _____
- ∞ HABIT TRACKER, Day ___ of 30

Wellbeing ACTIONS

- ☐ Today, I GET to _____ for me (prompts: JOY-FULL List p.15)
- ☐ Today, I GET to _____ my baby.
- ☐ Today, I GET to _____ for/with _____
  (e.g., spouse, kids, friends)

Nighttime REFLECTION

- ∞ WIN: I am _Celebrating_ myself for _____
- ∞ CHALLENGE: It felt hard when _____
  - ♥ I choose to see this as an opportunity to _____
  - ♥ Say aloud: *I forgive, and I release this challenge with love. *Inhale, Exhale**
- ∞ SUPPORT: I felt supported today by/when _____
  _____
- ∞ GRATITUDE: I am grateful for _____
  _____
- ∞ INTENTION: My intention for the morning is _____

Saturday

Morning PEP TALK

- ∞ In the mirror, with one hand on your heart: I LOVE YOU. YOU'VE GOT THIS, _____!
  (NAME)
- ∞ Affirmation: I (AM) _____
- ∞ I am grateful for (3+) _____
  _____
- ∞ I thank my body for _____
- ∞ HABIT TRACKER, Day ___ of 30

Wellbeing ACTIONS

- ☐ Today, I GET to _____ for me (prompts: JOY-FULL List p.15)
- ☐ Today, I GET to _____ my baby.
- ☐ Today, I GET to _____ for/with _____
  (e.g., spouse, kids, friends)

Nighttime REFLECTION

- ∞ WIN: I am *Celebrating* myself for _____
- ∞ CHALLENGE: It felt hard when _____
    - ♥ I choose to see this as an opportunity to _____
    - ♥ Say aloud: *I forgive, and I release this challenge with love. *Inhale, Exhale**
- ∞ SUPPORT: I felt supported today by/when _____
  _____
- ∞ GRATITUDE: I am grateful for _____
  _____
- ∞ INTENTION: My intention for the morning is _____

Sunday

Morning PEP TALK

- ∞ In the mirror, with one hand on your heart: I LOVE YOU. YOU'VE GOT THIS, _____!
  (NAME)
- ∞ Affirmation: I (AM) _____
- ∞ I am grateful for (3+) _____
  _____
- ∞ I thank my body for _____
- ∞ HABIT TRACKER, Day ___ of 30

Wellbeing ACTIONS

- ☐ Today, I GET to _____ for me (prompts: JOY-FULL List p.15)
- ☐ Today, I GET to _____ my baby.
- ☐ Today, I GET to _____ for/with _____
  (e.g., spouse, kids, friends)

Nighttime REFLECTION

- ∞ WIN: I am _Celebrating_ myself for _____
- ∞ CHALLENGE: It felt hard when _____
  - ♥ I choose to see this as an opportunity to _____
  - ♥ Say aloud: *I forgive, and I release this challenge with love. *Inhale, Exhale**
- ∞ SUPPORT: I felt supported today by/when _____
  _____
- ∞ GRATITUDE: I am grateful for _____
  _____
- ∞ INTENTION: My intention for the morning is _____

What's happening this week

Week of: _____

- ♥ Affirmation: I _____

- ♥ I will show myself grace this week by _____

- ♥ I am looking forward to _____

- ♥ I get to ask for support with _____

  By (action step) _____

- ☐ Review #2-6 from the Monthly Wellbeing Check-in. Take a moment to visualize yourself integrating these feelings, actions, and thoughts now, as well as throughout this week.

- ☐ Review upcoming appointments and set an alarm in your phone as needed.

Grocery list:
(TIP: Record here and take a picture to bring ease to the next grocery store trip.)

_____   _____   _____

_____   _____   _____

_____   _____   _____

_____   _____   _____

_____   _____   _____

_____   _____   _____

_____   _____   _____

_____   _____   _____

Monday

Morning PEP TALK

- ∞ In the mirror, with one hand on your heart: I LOVE YOU. YOU'VE GOT THIS, _____!
  (NAME)
- ∞ Affirmation: I (AM) _____
- ∞ I am grateful for (3+) _____
  _____
- ∞ I thank my body for _____
- ∞ HABIT TRACKER, Day ___ of 30

Wellbeing ACTIONS

- ☐ Today, I GET to _____ for me (prompts: JOY-FULL List p.15)
- ☐ Today, I GET to _____ my baby.
- ☐ Today, I GET to _____ for/with _____
  (e.g., spouse, kids, friends)

Nighttime REFLECTION

- ∞ WIN: I am <u>Celebrating</u> myself for _____
- ∞ CHALLENGE: It felt hard when _____
  - ♥ I choose to see this as an opportunity to _____
  - ♥ Say aloud: *I forgive, and I release this challenge with love.* *Inhale, Exhale*
- ∞ SUPPORT: I felt supported today by/when _____
  _____
- ∞ GRATITUDE: I am grateful for _____
  _____
- ∞ INTENTION: My intention for the morning is _____

Tuesday

Morning PEP TALK

- ∞ In the mirror, with one hand on your heart: I LOVE YOU. YOU'VE GOT THIS, _____!
   (NAME)
- ∞ Affirmation: I (AM) _____
- ∞ I am grateful for (3+) _____
  _____
- ∞ I thank my body for _____
- ∞ HABIT TRACKER, Day ___ of 30

Wellbeing ACTIONS

- ☐ Today, I GET to _____ for me (prompts: JOY-FULL List p.15)
- ☐ Today, I GET to _____ my baby.
- ☐ Today, I GET to _____ for/with _____
   (e.g., spouse, kids, friends)

Nighttime REFLECTION

- ∞ WIN: I am _Celebrating_ myself for _____
- ∞ CHALLENGE: It felt hard when _____
   - ♥ I choose to see this as an opportunity to _____
   - ♥ Say aloud: *I forgive, and I release this challenge with love.* *Inhale, Exhale*
- ∞ SUPPORT: I felt supported today by/when _____
  _____
- ∞ GRATITUDE: I am grateful for _____
  _____
- ∞ INTENTION: My intention for the morning is _____

Wednesday

Morning PEP TALK

- ∞ In the mirror, with one hand on your heart: I LOVE YOU. YOU'VE GOT THIS, _____!
  (NAME)
- ∞ Affirmation: I (AM) _____
- ∞ I am grateful for (3+) _____
  _____
- ∞ I thank my body for _____
- ∞ HABIT TRACKER, Day ___ of 30

Wellbeing ACTIONS

- ☐ Today, I GET to _____ for me (prompts: JOY-FULL List p.15)
- ☐ Today, I GET to _____ my baby.
- ☐ Today, I GET to _____ for/with _____
  (e.g., spouse, kids, friends)

Nighttime REFLECTION

- ∞ WIN: I am *Celebrating* myself for _____
- ∞ CHALLENGE: It felt hard when _____
  - ♥ I choose to see this as an opportunity to _____
  - ♥ Say aloud: *I forgive, and I release this challenge with love. *Inhale, Exhale**
- ∞ SUPPORT: I felt supported today by/when _____
  _____
- ∞ GRATITUDE: I am grateful for _____
  _____
- ∞ INTENTION: My intention for the morning is _____

Thursday

Morning PEP TALK

- ∞ In the mirror, with one hand on your heart: I LOVE YOU. YOU'VE GOT THIS, _____!

(NAME)
- ∞ Affirmation: I (AM) _____
- ∞ I am grateful for (3+) _____
  _____
- ∞ I thank my body for _____
- ∞ HABIT TRACKER, Day ___ of 30

Wellbeing ACTIONS

- ☐ Today, I GET to _____ for me (prompts: JOY-FULL List p.15)
- ☐ Today, I GET to _____ my baby.
- ☐ Today, I GET to _____ for/with _____

(e.g., spouse, kids, friends)

Nighttime REFLECTION

- ∞ WIN: I am *Celebrating* myself for _____
- ∞ CHALLENGE: It felt hard when _____
  - ♥ I choose to see this as an opportunity to _____
  - ♥ Say aloud: *I forgive, and I release this challenge with love. *Inhale, Exhale**
- ∞ SUPPORT: I felt supported today by/when _____
  _____
- ∞ GRATITUDE: I am grateful for _____
  _____
- ∞ INTENTION: My intention for the morning is _____

Friday

Morning PEP TALK

- ∞ In the mirror, with one hand on your heart: I LOVE YOU. YOU'VE GOT THIS, _____!
  (NAME)
- ∞ Affirmation: I (AM) _____
- ∞ I am grateful for (3+) _____
  _____
- ∞ I thank my body for _____
- ∞ HABIT TRACKER, Day ___ of 30

Wellbeing ACTIONS

- ☐ Today, I GET to _____ for me (prompts: JOY-FULL List p.15)
- ☐ Today, I GET to _____ my baby.
- ☐ Today, I GET to _____ for/with _____
  (e.g., spouse, kids, friends)

Nighttime REFLECTION

- ∞ WIN: I am *Celebrating* myself for _____
- ∞ CHALLENGE: It felt hard when _____
  - ♥ I choose to see this as an opportunity to _____
  - ♥ Say aloud: *I forgive, and I release this challenge with love. *Inhale, Exhale**
- ∞ SUPPORT: I felt supported today by/when _____
  _____
- ∞ GRATITUDE: I am grateful for _____
  _____
- ∞ INTENTION: My intention for the morning is _____

Saturday

Morning PEP TALK

- ∞ In the mirror, with one hand on your heart: I LOVE YOU. YOU'VE GOT THIS, _____!
  (NAME)
- ∞ Affirmation: I (AM) _____
- ∞ I am grateful for (3+) _____
  _____
- ∞ I thank my body for _____
- ∞ HABIT TRACKER, Day ___ of 30

Wellbeing ACTIONS

- ☐ Today, I GET to _____ for me (prompts: JOY-FULL List p.15)
- ☐ Today, I GET to _____ my baby.
- ☐ Today, I GET to _____ for/with _____
  (e.g., spouse, kids, friends)

Nighttime REFLECTION

- ∞ WIN: I am *Celebrating* myself for _____
- ∞ CHALLENGE: It felt hard when _____
  - ♥ I choose to see this as an opportunity to _____
  - ♥ Say aloud: *I forgive, and I release this challenge with love. *Inhale, Exhale**
- ∞ SUPPORT: I felt supported today by/when _____
  _____
- ∞ GRATITUDE: I am grateful for _____
  _____
- ∞ INTENTION: My intention for the morning is _____

Sunday

Morning PEP TALK

- ∞ In the mirror, with one hand on your heart: I LOVE YOU. YOU'VE GOT THIS, _____!
  (NAME)
- ∞ Affirmation: I (AM) _____
- ∞ I am grateful for (3+) _____
  _____
- ∞ I thank my body for _____
- ∞ HABIT TRACKER, Day ___ of 30

Wellbeing ACTIONS

- ☐ Today, I GET to _____ for me (prompts: JOY-FULL List p.15)
- ☐ Today, I GET to _____ my baby.
- ☐ Today, I GET to _____ for/with _____
  (e.g., spouse, kids, friends)

Nighttime REFLECTION

- ∞ WIN: I am *Celebrating* myself for _____
- ∞ CHALLENGE: It felt hard when _____
  - ♥ I choose to see this as an opportunity to _____
  - ♥ Say aloud: *I forgive, and I release this challenge with love.* *Inhale, Exhale*
- ∞ SUPPORT: I felt supported today by/when _____
  _____
- ∞ GRATITUDE: I am grateful for _____
  _____
- ∞ INTENTION: My intention for the morning is _____

What's happening this week

Week of: _____

- ♥ Affirmation: I _____
- ♥ I will show myself grace this week by _____
- ♥ I am looking forward to _____
- ♥ I get to ask for support with _____

      By (action step) _____

- ☐ Review #2-6 from the Monthly Wellbeing Check-in. Take a moment to visualize yourself integrating these feelings, actions, and thoughts now, as well as throughout this week.

- ☐ Review upcoming appointments and set an alarm in your phone as needed.

Grocery list:
(TIP: Record here and take a picture to bring ease to the next grocery store trip.)

_____	_____	_____
_____	_____	_____
_____	_____	_____
_____	_____	_____
_____	_____	_____
_____	_____	_____
_____	_____	_____

<u>Monday</u>

Morning PEP TALK

- ∞ In the mirror, with one hand on your heart: I LOVE YOU. YOU'VE GOT THIS, _____!
  (NAME)
- ∞ Affirmation: I (AM) _____
- ∞ I am grateful for (3+) _____
  _____
- ∞ I thank my body for _____
- ∞ HABIT TRACKER, Day ___ of 30

Wellbeing ACTIONS

- ☐ Today, I GET to _____ for me (prompts: JOY-FULL List p.15)
- ☐ Today, I GET to _____ my baby.
- ☐ Today, I GET to _____ for/with _____
  (e.g., spouse, kids, friends)

Nighttime REFLECTION

- ∞ WIN: I am <u>Celebrating</u> myself for _____
- ∞ CHALLENGE: It felt hard when _____
  - ♥ I choose to see this as an opportunity to _____
  - ♥ Say aloud: *I forgive, and I release this challenge with love.*
    Inhale, Exhale
- ∞ SUPPORT: I felt supported today by/when _____
  _____
- ∞ GRATITUDE: I am grateful for _____
  _____
- ∞ INTENTION: My intention for the morning is _____

Tuesday

Morning PEP TALK

- ∞ In the mirror, with one hand on your heart: I LOVE YOU. YOU'VE GOT THIS, _____!
  (NAME)
- ∞ Affirmation: I (AM) _____
- ∞ I am grateful for (3+) _____
  _____
- ∞ I thank my body for _____
- ∞ HABIT TRACKER, Day ___ of 30

Wellbeing ACTIONS

- ☐ Today, I GET to _____ for me (prompts: JOY-FULL List p.15)
- ☐ Today, I GET to _____ my baby.
- ☐ Today, I GET to _____ for/with _____
  (e.g., spouse, kids, friends)

Nighttime REFLECTION

- ∞ WIN: I am <u>Celebrating</u> myself for _____
- ∞ CHALLENGE: It felt hard when _____
  - ♥ I choose to see this as an opportunity to _____
  - ♥ Say aloud: *I forgive, and I release this challenge with love. *Inhale, Exhale**
- ∞ SUPPORT: I felt supported today by/when _____
  _____
- ∞ GRATITUDE: I am grateful for _____
  _____
- ∞ INTENTION: My intention for the morning is _____

Wednesday

Morning PEP TALK

- ∞ In the mirror, with one hand on your heart: I LOVE YOU. YOU'VE GOT THIS, _____!
  (NAME)
- ∞ Affirmation: I (AM) _____
- ∞ I am grateful for (3+) _____
  _____
- ∞ I thank my body for _____
- ∞ HABIT TRACKER, Day ___ of 30

Wellbeing ACTIONS

- ☐ Today, I GET to _____ for me (prompts: JOY-FULL List p.15)
- ☐ Today, I GET to _____ my baby.
- ☐ Today, I GET to _____ for/with _____
  (e.g., spouse, kids, friends)

Nighttime REFLECTION

- ∞ WIN: I am <u>Celebrating</u> myself for _____
- ∞ CHALLENGE: It felt hard when _____
  - ♥ I choose to see this as an opportunity to _____
  - ♥ Say aloud: *I forgive, and I release this challenge with love.* *Inhale, Exhale*
- ∞ SUPPORT: I felt supported today by/when _____
  _____
- ∞ GRATITUDE: I am grateful for _____
  _____
- ∞ INTENTION: My intention for the morning is _____

Thursday

Morning PEP TALK

- ∞ In the mirror, with one hand on your heart: I LOVE YOU. YOU'VE GOT THIS, _____!

(NAME)
- ∞ Affirmation: I (AM) _____
- ∞ I am grateful for (3+) _____
  _____
- ∞ I thank my body for _____
- ∞ HABIT TRACKER, Day ___ of 30

Wellbeing ACTIONS

- ☐ Today, I GET to _____ for me (prompts: JOY-FULL List p.15)
- ☐ Today, I GET to _____ my baby.
- ☐ Today, I GET to _____ for/with _____

(e.g., spouse, kids, friends)

Nighttime REFLECTION

- ∞ WIN: I am *Celebrating* myself for _____
- ∞ CHALLENGE: It felt hard when _____
  - ♥ I choose to see this as an opportunity to _____
  - ♥ Say aloud: *I forgive, and I release this challenge with love. *Inhale, Exhale**
- ∞ SUPPORT: I felt supported today by/when _____
  _____
- ∞ GRATITUDE: I am grateful for _____
  _____
- ∞ INTENTION: My intention for the morning is _____

Friday

Morning PEP TALK

- ∞ In the mirror, with one hand on your heart: I LOVE YOU. YOU'VE GOT THIS, _____!
  (NAME)
- ∞ Affirmation: I (AM) _____
- ∞ I am grateful for (3+) _____
  _____
- ∞ I thank my body for _____
- ∞ HABIT TRACKER, Day ___ of 30

Wellbeing ACTIONS

- ☐ Today, I GET to _____ for me (prompts: JOY-FULL List p.15)
- ☐ Today, I GET to _____ my baby.
- ☐ Today, I GET to _____ for/with _____
  (e.g., spouse, kids, friends)

Nighttime REFLECTION

- ∞ WIN: I am <u>Celebrating</u> myself for _____
- ∞ CHALLENGE: It felt hard when _____
  - ♥ I choose to see this as an opportunity to _____
  - ♥ Say aloud: *I forgive, and I release this challenge with love. *Inhale, Exhale**
- ∞ SUPPORT: I felt supported today by/when _____
  _____
- ∞ GRATITUDE: I am grateful for _____
  _____
- ∞ INTENTION: My intention for the morning is _____

Saturday

Morning PEP TALK

- ∞ In the mirror, with one hand on your heart: I LOVE YOU. YOU'VE GOT THIS, _____!
  (NAME)
- ∞ Affirmation: I (AM) _____
- ∞ I am grateful for (3+) _____
  _____
- ∞ I thank my body for _____
- ∞ HABIT TRACKER, Day ___ of 30

Wellbeing ACTIONS

- ☐ Today, I GET to _____ for me (prompts: JOY-FULL List p.15)
- ☐ Today, I GET to _____ my baby.
- ☐ Today, I GET to _____ for/with _____
  (e.g., spouse, kids, friends)

Nighttime REFLECTION

- ∞ WIN: I am <u>Celebrating</u> myself for _____
- ∞ CHALLENGE: It felt hard when _____
  - ♥ I choose to see this as an opportunity to _____
  - ♥ Say aloud: *I forgive, and I release this challenge with love. *Inhale, Exhale**
- ∞ SUPPORT: I felt supported today by/when _____
  _____
- ∞ GRATITUDE: I am grateful for _____
  _____
- ∞ INTENTION: My intention for the morning is _____

<u>Sunday</u>

Morning PEP TALK

- ∞ In the mirror, with one hand on your heart: I LOVE YOU. YOU'VE GOT THIS, _____!

(NAME)
- ∞ Affirmation: I (AM) _____
- ∞ I am grateful for (3+) _____
  _____
- ∞ I thank my body for _____
- ∞ HABIT TRACKER, Day ___ of 30

Wellbeing ACTIONS

- ☐ Today, I GET to _____ for me (prompts: JOY-FULL List p.15)
- ☐ Today, I GET to _____ my baby.
- ☐ Today, I GET to _____ for/with _____

(e.g., spouse, kids, friends)

Nighttime REFLECTION

- ∞ WIN: I am <u>Celebrating</u> myself for _____
- ∞ CHALLENGE: It felt hard when _____
    - ♥ I choose to see this as an opportunity to _____
    - ♥ Say aloud: *I forgive, and I release this challenge with love. *Inhale, Exhale**
- ∞ SUPPORT: I felt supported today by/when _____
  _____
- ∞ GRATITUDE: I am grateful for _____
  _____
- ∞ INTENTION: My intention for the morning is _____

Monthly Recap

- ♥ I am Celebrating _____!
    - ◊ In my head, I feel _____
    - ◊ In my heart, I feel _____
    - ◊ In my body, I feel _____
- ♥ My favourite activities this month were _____
_____
    - because _____
- ♥ My favourite affirmations this month were _____
_____
    - because _____
- ♥ It felt hard when _____
    - From this, I learned _____
- ♥ I feel more joy and ease in my life when I _____
_____
- ♥ I felt most supported this month when _____
- ♥ I am grateful for _____
- ♥ The boundary I set up at the beginning of the month helped me by
_____
- ♥ I am celebrating my new habit this month!
    - I am bringing this new habit with me into next month because (impact)
_____
- ♥ Special milestones/memories (date and event):

MONTH:

Free write/Notes/Lessons/Draw

MONTH: _____

SUNDAY	MONDAY	TUESDAY	WEDNESDAY
___	___	___	___
___	___	___	___
___	___	___	___
___	___	___	___
___	___	___	___

Record special dates, appointments, milestones, etc.

THURSDAY	FRIDAY	SATURDAY	NOTES
___	___	___	
___	___	___	
___	___	___	
___	___	___	
___	___	___	

Monthly Wellbeing Check-in

MONTH: _____

1. How do I feel right now?

    ◊ In my head (mentally): _____
       _____

    ◊ In my heart (emotionally): _____
       _____

    ◊ In my body (physically): _____
       _____

2. How do I desire to feel?

    ◊ In my head (mentally): _____
       _____

    ◊ In my heart (emotionally): _____
       _____

    ◊ In my body (physically): _____
       _____

3. What actions can I take to help me feel the way I described above? What thoughts can I have to help me feel this way?

    ◊ In my head (mentally): _____
       _____

    ◊ In my heart (emotionally): _____
       _____

    ◊ In my body (physically): _____
       _____

4. What am I excited for this month? _____

_____

5. What boundary am I setting up this month? _____

_____

    ◊   Action(s) to set up this boundary: _____

        _____

6. HABIT TRACKER (e.g., action/thought you wrote about for your desired feeling in #3):

I _____ am developing the habit of _____ this month.
   (NAME)

Picture this as a habit already. How do I feel? How am I showing up? What is different?

_____

_____

_____

_____

_____

_____

I understand that I may miss a day. I will show myself grace and re-commit the next day.

This habit supports me.

I am doing my best and I am Thriving!

What's happening this week

Week of: _____

- ♥ Affirmation: I _____

- ♥ I will show myself grace this week by _____

- ♥ I am looking forward to _____

- ♥ I get to ask for support with _____

    By (action step) _____

- ☐ Review #2-6 from the Monthly Wellbeing Check-in. Take a moment to visualize yourself integrating these feelings, actions, and thoughts now, as well as throughout this week.

- ☐ Review upcoming appointments and set an alarm in your phone as needed.

Grocery list:
(TIP: Record here and take a picture to bring ease to the next grocery store trip.)

Monday

Morning PEP TALK

- ∞ In the mirror, with one hand on your heart: I LOVE YOU. YOU'VE GOT THIS, _____!

(NAME)
- ∞ Affirmation: I (AM) _____
- ∞ I am grateful for (3+) _____
  _____
- ∞ I thank my body for _____
- ∞ HABIT TRACKER, Day ___ of 30

Wellbeing ACTIONS

- ☐ Today, I GET to _____ for me (prompts: JOY-FULL List p.15)
- ☐ Today, I GET to _____ my baby.
- ☐ Today, I GET to _____ for/with _____

(e.g., spouse, kids, friends)

Nighttime REFLECTION

- ∞ WIN: I am _Celebrating_ myself for _____
- ∞ CHALLENGE: It felt hard when _____
  - ♥ I choose to see this as an opportunity to _____
  - ♥ Say aloud: *I forgive, and I release this challenge with love.* *Inhale, Exhale*
- ∞ SUPPORT: I felt supported today by/when _____
  _____
- ∞ GRATITUDE: I am grateful for _____
  _____
- ∞ INTENTION: My intention for the morning is _____

Tuesday

Morning PEP TALK

∞ In the mirror, with one hand on your heart: I LOVE YOU. YOU'VE GOT THIS, _____!
(NAME)

∞ Affirmation: I (AM) _____

∞ I am grateful for (3+) _____
_____

∞ I thank my body for _____

∞ HABIT TRACKER, Day ___ of 30

Wellbeing ACTIONS

☐ Today, I GET to _____ for me (prompts: JOY-FULL List p.15)

☐ Today, I GET to _____ my baby.

☐ Today, I GET to _____ for/with _____
(e.g., spouse, kids, friends)

Nighttime REFLECTION

∞ WIN: I am <u>Celebrating</u> myself for _____

∞ CHALLENGE: It felt hard when _____

    ♥ I choose to see this as an opportunity to _____

    ♥ Say aloud: *I forgive, and I release this challenge with love. *Inhale, Exhale**

∞ SUPPORT: I felt supported today by/when _____
_____

∞ GRATITUDE: I am grateful for _____
_____

∞ INTENTION: My intention for the morning is _____

Wednesday

Morning PEP TALK

- ∞ In the mirror, with one hand on your heart: I LOVE YOU. YOU'VE GOT THIS, _____!
  (NAME)
- ∞ Affirmation: I (AM) _____
- ∞ I am grateful for (3+) _____
  _____
- ∞ I thank my body for _____
- ∞ HABIT TRACKER, Day ___ of 30

Wellbeing ACTIONS

- ☐ Today, I GET to _____ for me (prompts: JOY-FULL List p.15)
- ☐ Today, I GET to _____ my baby.
- ☐ Today, I GET to _____ for/with _____
  (e.g., spouse, kids, friends)

Nighttime REFLECTION

- ∞ WIN: I am *Celebrating* myself for _____
- ∞ CHALLENGE: It felt hard when _____
  - ♥ I choose to see this as an opportunity to _____
  - ♥ Say aloud: *I forgive, and I release this challenge with love. *Inhale, Exhale**
- ∞ SUPPORT: I felt supported today by/when _____
  _____
- ∞ GRATITUDE: I am grateful for _____
  _____
- ∞ INTENTION: My intention for the morning is _____

Thursday

Morning PEP TALK

- ∞ In the mirror, with one hand on your heart: I LOVE YOU. YOU'VE GOT THIS, _____!

(NAME)
- ∞ Affirmation: I (AM) _____
- ∞ I am grateful for (3+) _____
  _____
- ∞ I thank my body for _____
- ∞ HABIT TRACKER, Day ___ of 30

Wellbeing ACTIONS

- ☐ Today, I GET to _____ for me (prompts: JOY-FULL List p.15)
- ☐ Today, I GET to _____ my baby.
- ☐ Today, I GET to _____ for/with _____

(e.g., spouse, kids, friends)

Nighttime REFLECTION

- ∞ WIN: I am _Celebrating_ myself for _____
- ∞ CHALLENGE: It felt hard when _____
  - ♥ I choose to see this as an opportunity to _____
  - ♥ Say aloud: *I forgive, and I release this challenge with love.* *Inhale, Exhale*
- ∞ SUPPORT: I felt supported today by/when _____
  _____
- ∞ GRATITUDE: I am grateful for _____
  _____
- ∞ INTENTION: My intention for the morning is _____

<u>Friday</u>

Morning PEP TALK

- ∞ In the mirror, with one hand on your heart: I LOVE YOU. YOU'VE GOT THIS, _____!
  (NAME)
- ∞ Affirmation: I (AM) _____
- ∞ I am grateful for (3+) _____
  _____
- ∞ I thank my body for _____
- ∞ HABIT TRACKER, Day ___ of 30

Wellbeing ACTIONS

- ☐ Today, I GET to _____ for me (prompts: JOY-FULL List p.15)
- ☐ Today, I GET to _____ my baby.
- ☐ Today, I GET to _____ for/with _____
  (e.g., spouse, kids, friends)

Nighttime REFLECTION

- ∞ WIN: I am <u>*Celebrating*</u> myself for _____
- ∞ CHALLENGE: It felt hard when _____
  - ♥ I choose to see this as an opportunity to _____
  - ♥ Say aloud: *I forgive, and I release this challenge with love. *Inhale, Exhale**
- ∞ SUPPORT: I felt supported today by/when _____
  _____
- ∞ GRATITUDE: I am grateful for _____
  _____
- ∞ INTENTION: My intention for the morning is _____

Saturday

Morning PEP TALK

- ∞ In the mirror, with one hand on your heart: I LOVE YOU. YOU'VE GOT THIS, _____!
  (NAME)
- ∞ Affirmation: I (AM) _____
- ∞ I am grateful for (3+) _____
  _____
- ∞ I thank my body for _____
- ∞ HABIT TRACKER, Day ___ of 30

Wellbeing ACTIONS

- ☐ Today, I GET to _____ for me (prompts: JOY-FULL List p.15)
- ☐ Today, I GET to _____ my baby.
- ☐ Today, I GET to _____ for/with _____
  (e.g., spouse, kids, friends)

Nighttime REFLECTION

- ∞ WIN: I am *Celebrating* myself for _____
- ∞ CHALLENGE: It felt hard when _____
  - ♥ I choose to see this as an opportunity to _____
  - ♥ Say aloud: *I forgive, and I release this challenge with love. *Inhale, Exhale**
- ∞ SUPPORT: I felt supported today by/when _____
  _____
- ∞ GRATITUDE: I am grateful for _____
  _____
- ∞ INTENTION: My intention for the morning is _____

Sunday

Morning PEP TALK

- ∞ In the mirror, with one hand on your heart: I LOVE YOU. YOU'VE GOT THIS, _____!
  (NAME)
- ∞ Affirmation: I (AM) _____
- ∞ I am grateful for (3+) _____
  _____
- ∞ I thank my body for _____
- ∞ HABIT TRACKER, Day ___ of 30

Wellbeing ACTIONS

- ☐ Today, I GET to _____ for me (prompts: JOY-FULL List p.15)
- ☐ Today, I GET to _____ my baby.
- ☐ Today, I GET to _____ for/with _____
  (e.g., spouse, kids, friends)

Nighttime REFLECTION

- ∞ WIN: I am *Celebrating* myself for _____
- ∞ CHALLENGE: It felt hard when _____
  - ♥ I choose to see this as an opportunity to _____
  - ♥ Say aloud: *I forgive, and I release this challenge with love. *Inhale, Exhale**
- ∞ SUPPORT: I felt supported today by/when _____
  _____
- ∞ GRATITUDE: I am grateful for _____
  _____
- ∞ INTENTION: My intention for the morning is _____

What's happening this week

Week of: _____

- ♥ Affirmation: I _____
- ♥ I will show myself grace this week by _____
- ♥ I am looking forward to _____
- ♥ I get to ask for support with _____

　　　By (action step) _____

☐ Review #2-6 from the Monthly Wellbeing Check-in. Take a moment to visualize yourself integrating these feelings, actions, and thoughts now, as well as throughout this week.

☐ Review upcoming appointments and set an alarm in your phone as needed.

Grocery list:
(TIP: Record here and take a picture to bring ease to the next grocery store trip.)

_____　　_____　　_____
_____　　_____　　_____
_____　　_____　　_____
_____　　_____　　_____
_____　　_____　　_____
_____　　_____　　_____
_____　　_____　　_____

Monday

Morning PEP TALK

- ∞ In the mirror, with one hand on your heart: I LOVE YOU. YOU'VE GOT THIS, _____!
  (NAME)
- ∞ Affirmation: I (AM) _____
- ∞ I am grateful for (3+) _____
  _____
- ∞ I thank my body for _____
- ∞ HABIT TRACKER, Day ___ of 30

Wellbeing ACTIONS

- ☐ Today, I GET to _____ for me (prompts: JOY-FULL List p.15)
- ☐ Today, I GET to _____ my baby.
- ☐ Today, I GET to _____ for/with _____
  (e.g., spouse, kids, friends)

Nighttime REFLECTION

- ∞ WIN: I am <u>Celebrating</u> myself for _____
- ∞ CHALLENGE: It felt hard when _____
  - ♥ I choose to see this as an opportunity to _____
  - ♥ Say aloud: *I forgive, and I release this challenge with love.* *Inhale, Exhale*
- ∞ SUPPORT: I felt supported today by/when _____
  _____
- ∞ GRATITUDE: I am grateful for _____
  _____
- ∞ INTENTION: My intention for the morning is _____

Tuesday

Morning PEP TALK

- ∞ In the mirror, with one hand on your heart: I LOVE YOU. YOU'VE GOT THIS, _____!
  (NAME)
- ∞ Affirmation: I (AM) _____
- ∞ I am grateful for (3+) _____
  _____
- ∞ I thank my body for _____
- ∞ HABIT TRACKER, Day ___ of 30

Wellbeing ACTIONS

- ☐ Today, I GET to _____ for me (prompts: JOY-FULL List p.15)
- ☐ Today, I GET to _____ my baby.
- ☐ Today, I GET to _____ for/with _____
  (e.g., spouse, kids, friends)

Nighttime REFLECTION

- ∞ WIN: I am <u>Celebrating</u> myself for _____
- ∞ CHALLENGE: It felt hard when _____
  - ♥ I choose to see this as an opportunity to _____
  - ♥ Say aloud: *I forgive, and I release this challenge with love. *Inhale, Exhale**
- ∞ SUPPORT: I felt supported today by/when _____
  _____
- ∞ GRATITUDE: I am grateful for _____
  _____
- ∞ INTENTION: My intention for the morning is _____

Wednesday

Morning PEP TALK

- ∞ In the mirror, with one hand on your heart: I LOVE YOU. YOU'VE GOT THIS, _____!
(NAME)
- ∞ Affirmation: I (AM) _____
- ∞ I am grateful for (3+) _____
_____
- ∞ I thank my body for _____
- ∞ HABIT TRACKER, Day ___ of 30

Wellbeing ACTIONS

- ☐ Today, I GET to _____ for me (prompts: JOY-FULL List p.15)
- ☐ Today, I GET to _____ my baby.
- ☐ Today, I GET to _____ for/with _____
(e.g., spouse, kids, friends)

Nighttime REFLECTION

- ∞ WIN: I am *Celebrating* myself for _____
- ∞ CHALLENGE: It felt hard when _____
    - ♥ I choose to see this as an opportunity to _____
    - ♥ Say aloud: *I forgive, and I release this challenge with love.* *Inhale, Exhale*
- ∞ SUPPORT: I felt supported today by/when _____
_____
- ∞ GRATITUDE: I am grateful for _____
_____
- ∞ INTENTION: My intention for the morning is _____

Thursday

Morning PEP TALK

- ∞ In the mirror, with one hand on your heart: I LOVE YOU. YOU'VE GOT THIS, _____!
  (NAME)
- ∞ Affirmation: I (AM) _____
- ∞ I am grateful for (3+) _____
  _____
- ∞ I thank my body for _____
- ∞ HABIT TRACKER, Day ___ of 30

Wellbeing ACTIONS

- ☐ Today, I GET to _____ for me (prompts: JOY-FULL List p.15)
- ☐ Today, I GET to _____ my baby.
- ☐ Today, I GET to _____ for/with _____
  (e.g., spouse, kids, friends)

Nighttime REFLECTION

- ∞ WIN: I am _Celebrating_ myself for _____
- ∞ CHALLENGE: It felt hard when _____
  - ♥ I choose to see this as an opportunity to _____
  - ♥ Say aloud: *I forgive, and I release this challenge with love. *Inhale, Exhale**
- ∞ SUPPORT: I felt supported today by/when _____
  _____
- ∞ GRATITUDE: I am grateful for _____
  _____
- ∞ INTENTION: My intention for the morning is _____

Friday

Morning PEP TALK

- ∞ In the mirror, with one hand on your heart: I LOVE YOU. YOU'VE GOT THIS, _____!
  (NAME)
- ∞ Affirmation: I (AM) _____
- ∞ I am grateful for (3+) _____
  _____
- ∞ I thank my body for _____
- ∞ HABIT TRACKER, Day ___ of 30

Wellbeing ACTIONS

- ☐ Today, I GET to _____ for me (prompts: JOY-FULL List p.15)
- ☐ Today, I GET to _____ my baby.
- ☐ Today, I GET to _____ for/with _____
  (e.g., spouse, kids, friends)

Nighttime REFLECTION

- ∞ WIN: I am *Celebrating* myself for _____
- ∞ CHALLENGE: It felt hard when _____
  - ♥ I choose to see this as an opportunity to _____
  - ♥ Say aloud: *I forgive, and I release this challenge with love.*
    Inhale, Exhale
- ∞ SUPPORT: I felt supported today by/when _____
  _____
- ∞ GRATITUDE: I am grateful for _____
  _____
- ∞ INTENTION: My intention for the morning is _____

Saturday

Morning PEP TALK

- ∞ In the mirror, with one hand on your heart: I LOVE YOU. YOU'VE GOT THIS, _____ !
  (NAME)
- ∞ Affirmation: I (AM) _____
- ∞ I am grateful for (3+) _____
  _____
- ∞ I thank my body for _____
- ∞ HABIT TRACKER, Day ___ of 30

Wellbeing ACTIONS

- ☐ Today, I GET to _____ for me (prompts: JOY-FULL List p.15)
- ☐ Today, I GET to _____ my baby.
- ☐ Today, I GET to _____ for/with _____
  (e.g., spouse, kids, friends)

Nighttime REFLECTION

- ∞ WIN: I am <u>Celebrating</u> myself for _____
- ∞ CHALLENGE: It felt hard when _____
  - ♥ I choose to see this as an opportunity to _____
  - ♥ Say aloud: *I forgive, and I release this challenge with love. *Inhale, Exhale**
- ∞ SUPPORT: I felt supported today by/when _____
  _____
- ∞ GRATITUDE: I am grateful for _____
  _____
- ∞ INTENTION: My intention for the morning is _____

Sunday

Morning PEP TALK

- ∞ In the mirror, with one hand on your heart: I LOVE YOU. YOU'VE GOT THIS, _____!
  (NAME)
- ∞ Affirmation: I (AM) _____
- ∞ I am grateful for (3+) _____
  _____
- ∞ I thank my body for _____
- ∞ HABIT TRACKER, Day ___ of 30

Wellbeing ACTIONS

- ☐ Today, I GET to _____ for me (prompts: JOY-FULL List p.15)
- ☐ Today, I GET to _____ my baby.
- ☐ Today, I GET to _____ for/with _____
  (e.g., spouse, kids, friends)

Nighttime REFLECTION

- ∞ WIN: I am *Celebrating* myself for _____
- ∞ CHALLENGE: It felt hard when _____
  - ♥ I choose to see this as an opportunity to _____
  - ♥ Say aloud: *I forgive, and I release this challenge with love. *Inhale, Exhale**
- ∞ SUPPORT: I felt supported today by/when _____
  _____
- ∞ GRATITUDE: I am grateful for _____
  _____
- ∞ INTENTION: My intention for the morning is _____

What's happening this week

Week of: _____

- ♥ Affirmation: I _____
- ♥ I will show myself grace this week by _____
- ♥ I am looking forward to _____
- ♥ I get to ask for support with _____

      By (action step) _____

☐ Review #2-6 from the Monthly Wellbeing Check-in. Take a moment to visualize yourself integrating these feelings, actions, and thoughts now, as well as throughout this week.

☐ Review upcoming appointments and set an alarm in your phone as needed.

Grocery list:
(TIP: Record here and take a picture to bring ease to the next grocery store trip.)

_____ _____ _____

_____ _____ _____

_____ _____ _____

_____ _____ _____

_____ _____ _____

_____ _____ _____

_____ _____ _____

Monday

Morning PEP TALK

- ∞ In the mirror, with one hand on your heart: I LOVE YOU. YOU'VE GOT THIS, _____!
  (NAME)
- ∞ Affirmation: I (AM) _____
- ∞ I am grateful for (3+) _____
  _____
- ∞ I thank my body for _____
- ∞ HABIT TRACKER, Day ___ of 30

Wellbeing ACTIONS

- ☐ Today, I GET to _____ for me (prompts: JOY-FULL List p.15)
- ☐ Today, I GET to _____ my baby.
- ☐ Today, I GET to _____ for/with _____
  (e.g., spouse, kids, friends)

Nighttime REFLECTION

- ∞ WIN: I am <u>Celebrating</u> myself for _____
- ∞ CHALLENGE: It felt hard when _____
    - ♥ I choose to see this as an opportunity to _____
    - ♥ Say aloud: *I forgive, and I release this challenge with love. *Inhale, Exhale**
- ∞ SUPPORT: I felt supported today by/when _____
  _____
- ∞ GRATITUDE: I am grateful for _____
  _____
- ∞ INTENTION: My intention for the morning is _____

Tuesday

Morning PEP TALK

- ∞ In the mirror, with one hand on your heart: I LOVE YOU. YOU'VE GOT THIS, _____!
  (NAME)
- ∞ Affirmation: I (AM) _____
- ∞ I am grateful for (3+) _____
  _____
- ∞ I thank my body for _____
- ∞ HABIT TRACKER, Day ___ of 30

Wellbeing ACTIONS

- ☐ Today, I GET to _____ for me (prompts: JOY-FULL List p.15)
- ☐ Today, I GET to _____ my baby.
- ☐ Today, I GET to _____ for/with _____
  (e.g., spouse, kids, friends)

Nighttime REFLECTION

- ∞ WIN: I am *Celebrating* myself for _____
- ∞ CHALLENGE: It felt hard when _____
  - ♥ I choose to see this as an opportunity to _____
  - ♥ Say aloud: *I forgive, and I release this challenge with love. *Inhale, Exhale**
- ∞ SUPPORT: I felt supported today by/when _____
  _____
- ∞ GRATITUDE: I am grateful for _____
  _____
- ∞ INTENTION: My intention for the morning is _____

Wednesday

Morning PEP TALK

- ∞ In the mirror, with one hand on your heart: I LOVE YOU. YOU'VE GOT THIS, _____!
  (NAME)
- ∞ Affirmation: I (AM) _____
- ∞ I am grateful for (3+) _____
  _____
- ∞ I thank my body for _____
- ∞ HABIT TRACKER, Day ___ of 30

Wellbeing ACTIONS

- ☐ Today, I GET to _____ for me (prompts: JOY-FULL List p.15)
- ☐ Today, I GET to _____ my baby.
- ☐ Today, I GET to _____ for/with _____
  (e.g., spouse, kids, friends)

Nighttime REFLECTION

- ∞ WIN: I am *Celebrating* myself for _____
- ∞ CHALLENGE: It felt hard when _____
  - ♥ I choose to see this as an opportunity to _____
  - ♥ Say aloud: *I forgive, and I release this challenge with love.*
    Inhale, Exhale
- ∞ SUPPORT: I felt supported today by/when _____
  _____
- ∞ GRATITUDE: I am grateful for _____
  _____
- ∞ INTENTION: My intention for the morning is _____

Thursday

Morning PEP TALK

- In the mirror, with one hand on your heart: I LOVE YOU. YOU'VE GOT THIS, _____!
  (NAME)
- Affirmation: I (AM) _____
- I am grateful for (3+) _____
  _____
- I thank my body for _____
- HABIT TRACKER, Day ___ of 30

Wellbeing ACTIONS

- ☐ Today, I GET to _____ for me (prompts: JOY-FULL List p.15)
- ☐ Today, I GET to _____ my baby.
- ☐ Today, I GET to _____ for/with _____
  (e.g., spouse, kids, friends)

Nighttime REFLECTION

- WIN: I am *Celebrating* myself for _____
- CHALLENGE: It felt hard when _____
  - ♥ I choose to see this as an opportunity to _____
  - ♥ Say aloud: *I forgive, and I release this challenge with love. *Inhale, Exhale**
- SUPPORT: I felt supported today by/when _____
  _____
- GRATITUDE: I am grateful for _____
  _____
- INTENTION: My intention for the morning is _____

Friday
_____

Morning PEP TALK

- ∞ In the mirror, with one hand on your heart: I LOVE YOU. YOU'VE GOT THIS, _____!
  (NAME)
- ∞ Affirmation: I (AM) _____
- ∞ I am grateful for (3+) _____
  _____
- ∞ I thank my body for _____
- ∞ HABIT TRACKER, Day ___ of 30

Wellbeing ACTIONS

- ☐ Today, I GET to _____ for me (prompts: JOY-FULL List p.15)
- ☐ Today, I GET to _____ my baby.
- ☐ Today, I GET to _____ for/with _____
  (e.g., spouse, kids, friends)

Nighttime REFLECTION

- ∞ WIN: I am *Celebrating* myself for _____
- ∞ CHALLENGE: It felt hard when _____
  - ♥ I choose to see this as an opportunity to _____
  - ♥ Say aloud: *I forgive, and I release this challenge with love. *Inhale, Exhale**
- ∞ SUPPORT: I felt supported today by/when _____
  _____
- ∞ GRATITUDE: I am grateful for _____
  _____
- ∞ INTENTION: My intention for the morning is _____

Saturday

Morning PEP TALK

- ∞ In the mirror, with one hand on your heart: I LOVE YOU. YOU'VE GOT THIS, _____!
  (NAME)
- ∞ Affirmation: I (AM) _____
- ∞ I am grateful for (3+) _____
  _____
- ∞ I thank my body for _____
- ∞ HABIT TRACKER, Day ___ of 30

Wellbeing ACTIONS

- ☐ Today, I GET to _____ for me (prompts: JOY-FULL List p.15)
- ☐ Today, I GET to _____ my baby.
- ☐ Today, I GET to _____ for/with _____
  (e.g., spouse, kids, friends)

Nighttime REFLECTION

- ∞ WIN: I am <u>Celebrating</u> myself for _____
- ∞ CHALLENGE: It felt hard when _____
  - ♥ I choose to see this as an opportunity to _____
  - ♥ Say aloud: *I forgive, and I release this challenge with love. *Inhale, Exhale**
- ∞ SUPPORT: I felt supported today by/when _____
  _____
- ∞ GRATITUDE: I am grateful for _____
  _____
- ∞ INTENTION: My intention for the morning is _____

Sunday

Morning PEP TALK

- ∞ In the mirror, with one hand on your heart: I LOVE YOU. YOU'VE GOT THIS, _____!
  (NAME)
- ∞ Affirmation: I (AM) _____
- ∞ I am grateful for (3+) _____
  _____
- ∞ I thank my body for _____
- ∞ HABIT TRACKER, Day ___ of 30

Wellbeing ACTIONS

- ☐ Today, I GET to _____ for me (prompts: JOY-FULL List p.15)
- ☐ Today, I GET to _____ my baby.
- ☐ Today, I GET to _____ for/with _____
  (e.g., spouse, kids, friends)

Nighttime REFLECTION

- ∞ WIN: I am <u>Celebrating</u> myself for _____
- ∞ CHALLENGE: It felt hard when _____
  - ♥ I choose to see this as an opportunity to _____
  - ♥ Say aloud: *I forgive, and I release this challenge with love. *Inhale, Exhale**
- ∞ SUPPORT: I felt supported today by/when _____
  _____
- ∞ GRATITUDE: I am grateful for _____
  _____
- ∞ INTENTION: My intention for the morning is _____

What's happening this week

Week of: _____

- ♥ Affirmation: I _____

- ♥ I will show myself grace this week by _____

- ♥ I am looking forward to _____

- ♥ I get to ask for support with _____

    By (action step) _____

- ☐ Review #2-6 from the Monthly Wellbeing Check-in. Take a moment to visualize yourself integrating these feelings, actions, and thoughts now, as well as throughout this week.

- ☐ Review upcoming appointments and set an alarm in your phone as needed.

Grocery list:
(TIP: Record here and take a picture to bring ease to the next grocery store trip.)

_____	_____	_____
_____	_____	_____
_____	_____	_____
_____	_____	_____
_____	_____	_____
_____	_____	_____

Monday

Morning PEP TALK

- ∞ In the mirror, with one hand on your heart: I LOVE YOU. YOU'VE GOT THIS, _____!
  (NAME)
- ∞ Affirmation: I (AM) _____
- ∞ I am grateful for (3+) _____
  _____
- ∞ I thank my body for _____
- ∞ HABIT TRACKER, Day ___ of 30

Wellbeing ACTIONS

- ☐ Today, I GET to _____ for me (prompts: JOY-FULL List p.15)
- ☐ Today, I GET to _____ my baby.
- ☐ Today, I GET to _____ for/with _____
  (e.g., spouse, kids, friends)

Nighttime REFLECTION

- ∞ WIN: I am <u>Celebrating</u> myself for _____
- ∞ CHALLENGE: It felt hard when _____
  - ♥ I choose to see this as an opportunity to _____
  - ♥ Say aloud: *I forgive, and I release this challenge with love.* *Inhale, Exhale*
- ∞ SUPPORT: I felt supported today by/when _____
  _____
- ∞ GRATITUDE: I am grateful for _____
  _____
- ∞ INTENTION: My intention for the morning is _____

Tuesday

Morning PEP TALK

- ∞ In the mirror, with one hand on your heart: I LOVE YOU. YOU'VE GOT THIS, _____!
  (NAME)
- ∞ Affirmation: I (AM) _____
- ∞ I am grateful for (3+) _____
  _____
- ∞ I thank my body for _____
- ∞ HABIT TRACKER, Day ___ of 30

Wellbeing ACTIONS

- ☐ Today, I GET to _____ for me (prompts: JOY-FULL List p.15)
- ☐ Today, I GET to _____ my baby.
- ☐ Today, I GET to _____ for/with _____
  (e.g., spouse, kids, friends)

Nighttime REFLECTION

- ∞ WIN: I am <u>Celebrating</u> myself for _____
- ∞ CHALLENGE: It felt hard when _____
  - ♥ I choose to see this as an opportunity to _____
  - ♥ Say aloud: *I forgive, and I release this challenge with love. *Inhale, Exhale**
- ∞ SUPPORT: I felt supported today by/when _____
  _____
- ∞ GRATITUDE: I am grateful for _____
  _____
- ∞ INTENTION: My intention for the morning is _____

Wednesday

Morning PEP TALK

- ∞ In the mirror, with one hand on your heart: I LOVE YOU. YOU'VE GOT THIS, _____!
  (NAME)
- ∞ Affirmation: I (AM) _____
- ∞ I am grateful for (3+) _____
- ∞ I thank my body for _____
- ∞ HABIT TRACKER, Day ___ of 30

Wellbeing ACTIONS

- ☐ Today, I GET to _____ for me (prompts: JOY-FULL List p.15)
- ☐ Today, I GET to _____ my baby.
- ☐ Today, I GET to _____ for/with _____
  (e.g., spouse, kids, friends)

Nighttime REFLECTION

- ∞ WIN: I am <u>*Celebrating*</u> myself for _____
- ∞ CHALLENGE: It felt hard when _____
  - ♥ I choose to see this as an opportunity to _____
  - ♥ Say aloud: *I forgive, and I release this challenge with love. *Inhale, Exhale**
- ∞ SUPPORT: I felt supported today by/when _____
- ∞ GRATITUDE: I am grateful for _____
- ∞ INTENTION: My intention for the morning is _____

Thursday

Morning PEP TALK

- ∞ In the mirror, with one hand on your heart: I LOVE YOU. YOU'VE GOT THIS, _____!
  (NAME)
- ∞ Affirmation: I (AM) _____
- ∞ I am grateful for (3+) _____
  _____
- ∞ I thank my body for _____
- ∞ HABIT TRACKER, Day ___ of 30

Wellbeing ACTIONS

- ☐ Today, I GET to _____ for me (prompts: JOY-FULL List p.15)
- ☐ Today, I GET to _____ my baby.
- ☐ Today, I GET to _____ for/with _____
  (e.g., spouse, kids, friends)

Nighttime REFLECTION

- ∞ WIN: I am <u>Celebrating</u> myself for _____
- ∞ CHALLENGE: It felt hard when _____
  - ♥ I choose to see this as an opportunity to _____
  - ♥ Say aloud: *I forgive, and I release this challenge with love. *Inhale, Exhale**
- ∞ SUPPORT: I felt supported today by/when _____
  _____
- ∞ GRATITUDE: I am grateful for _____
  _____
- ∞ INTENTION: My intention for the morning is _____

Friday

Morning PEP TALK

- ∞ In the mirror, with one hand on your heart: I LOVE YOU. YOU'VE GOT THIS, _____!
  (NAME)
- ∞ Affirmation: I (AM) _____
- ∞ I am grateful for (3+) _____
  _____
- ∞ I thank my body for _____
- ∞ HABIT TRACKER, Day ___ of 30

Wellbeing ACTIONS

- ☐ Today, I GET to _____ for me (prompts: JOY-FULL List p.15)
- ☐ Today, I GET to _____ my baby.
- ☐ Today, I GET to _____ for/with _____
  (e.g., spouse, kids, friends)

Nighttime REFLECTION

- ∞ WIN: I am *Celebrating* myself for _____
- ∞ CHALLENGE: It felt hard when _____
  - ♥ I choose to see this as an opportunity to _____
  - ♥ Say aloud: *I forgive, and I release this challenge with love. *Inhale, Exhale**
- ∞ SUPPORT: I felt supported today by/when _____
  _____
- ∞ GRATITUDE: I am grateful for _____
  _____
- ∞ INTENTION: My intention for the morning is _____

Saturday

Morning PEP TALK

- ∞ In the mirror, with one hand on your heart: I LOVE YOU. YOU'VE GOT THIS, _____!
  (NAME)
- ∞ Affirmation: I (AM) _____
- ∞ I am grateful for (3+) _____
  _____
- ∞ I thank my body for _____
- ∞ HABIT TRACKER, Day ___ of 30

Wellbeing ACTIONS

- ☐ Today, I GET to _____ for me (prompts: JOY-FULL List p.15)
- ☐ Today, I GET to _____ my baby.
- ☐ Today, I GET to _____ for/with _____
  (e.g., spouse, kids, friends)

Nighttime REFLECTION

- ∞ WIN: I am <u>Celebrating</u> myself for _____
- ∞ CHALLENGE: It felt hard when _____
  - ♥ I choose to see this as an opportunity to _____
  - ♥ Say aloud: *I forgive, and I release this challenge with love. *Inhale, Exhale**
- ∞ SUPPORT: I felt supported today by/when _____
  _____
- ∞ GRATITUDE: I am grateful for _____
  _____
- ∞ INTENTION: My intention for the morning is _____

Sunday

Morning PEP TALK

- ∞ In the mirror, with one hand on your heart: I LOVE YOU. YOU'VE GOT THIS, _____!
  (NAME)
- ∞ Affirmation: I (AM) _____
- ∞ I am grateful for (3+) _____
  _____
- ∞ I thank my body for _____
- ∞ HABIT TRACKER, Day ___ of 30

Wellbeing ACTIONS

- ☐ Today, I GET to _____ for me (prompts: JOY-FULL List p.15)
- ☐ Today, I GET to _____ my baby.
- ☐ Today, I GET to _____ for/with _____
  (e.g., spouse, kids, friends)

Nighttime REFLECTION

- ∞ WIN: I am *Celebrating* myself for _____
- ∞ CHALLENGE: It felt hard when _____
  - ♥ I choose to see this as an opportunity to _____
  - ♥ Say aloud: *I forgive, and I release this challenge with love. *Inhale, Exhale**
- ∞ SUPPORT: I felt supported today by/when _____
  _____
- ∞ GRATITUDE: I am grateful for _____
  _____
- ∞ INTENTION: My intention for the morning is _____

What's happening this week

Week of: _____

- ♥ Affirmation: I _____
- ♥ I will show myself grace this week by _____
- ♥ I am looking forward to _____
- ♥ I get to ask for support with _____

    By (action step) _____

- ☐ Review #2-6 from the Monthly Wellbeing Check-in. Take a moment to visualize yourself integrating these feelings, actions, and thoughts now, as well as throughout this week.

- ☐ Review upcoming appointments and set an alarm in your phone as needed.

Grocery list:
(TIP: Record here and take a picture to bring ease to the next grocery store trip.)

_____	_____	_____
_____	_____	_____
_____	_____	_____
_____	_____	_____
_____	_____	_____
_____	_____	_____
_____	_____	_____

Monday

Morning PEP TALK

- ∞ In the mirror, with one hand on your heart: I LOVE YOU. YOU'VE GOT THIS, _____!
  (NAME)
- ∞ Affirmation: I (AM) _____
- ∞ I am grateful for (3+) _____
  _____
- ∞ I thank my body for _____
- ∞ HABIT TRACKER, Day ___ of 30

Wellbeing ACTIONS

- ☐ Today, I GET to _____ for me (prompts: JOY-FULL List p.15)
- ☐ Today, I GET to _____ my baby.
- ☐ Today, I GET to _____ for/with _____
  (e.g., spouse, kids, friends)

Nighttime REFLECTION

- ∞ WIN: I am <u>Celebrating</u> myself for _____
- ∞ CHALLENGE: It felt hard when _____
  - ♥ I choose to see this as an opportunity to _____
  - ♥ Say aloud: *I forgive, and I release this challenge with love. *Inhale, Exhale**
- ∞ SUPPORT: I felt supported today by/when _____
  _____
- ∞ GRATITUDE: I am grateful for _____
  _____
- ∞ INTENTION: My intention for the morning is _____

Tuesday

Morning PEP TALK

- ∞ In the mirror, with one hand on your heart: I LOVE YOU. YOU'VE GOT THIS, _____ !

(NAME)
- ∞ Affirmation: I (AM) _____
- ∞ I am grateful for (3+) _____
  _____
- ∞ I thank my body for _____
- ∞ HABIT TRACKER, Day ___ of 30

Wellbeing ACTIONS

- ☐ Today, I GET to _____ for me (prompts: JOY-FULL List p.15)
- ☐ Today, I GET to _____ my baby.
- ☐ Today, I GET to _____ for/with _____

(e.g., spouse, kids, friends)

Nighttime REFLECTION

- ∞ WIN: I am _Celebrating_ myself for _____
- ∞ CHALLENGE: It felt hard when _____
    - ♥ I choose to see this as an opportunity to _____
    - ♥ Say aloud: *I forgive, and I release this challenge with love. *Inhale, Exhale**
- ∞ SUPPORT: I felt supported today by/when _____
  _____
- ∞ GRATITUDE: I am grateful for _____
  _____
- ∞ INTENTION: My intention for the morning is _____

Wednesday

Morning PEP TALK

- ∞ In the mirror, with one hand on your heart: I LOVE YOU. YOU'VE GOT THIS, _____!
    (NAME)
- ∞ Affirmation: I (AM) _____
- ∞ I am grateful for (3+) _____
  _____
- ∞ I thank my body for _____
- ∞ HABIT TRACKER, Day ___ of 30

Wellbeing ACTIONS

- ☐ Today, I GET to _____ for me (prompts: JOY-FULL List p.15)
- ☐ Today, I GET to _____ my baby.
- ☐ Today, I GET to _____ for/with _____
    (e.g., spouse, kids, friends)

Nighttime REFLECTION

- ∞ WIN: I am <u>Celebrating</u> myself for _____
- ∞ CHALLENGE: It felt hard when _____
    - ♥ I choose to see this as an opportunity to _____
    - ♥ Say aloud: *I forgive, and I release this challenge with love. *Inhale, Exhale**
- ∞ SUPPORT: I felt supported today by/when _____
  _____
- ∞ GRATITUDE: I am grateful for _____
  _____
- ∞ INTENTION: My intention for the morning is _____

Thursday

Morning PEP TALK

- ∞ In the mirror, with one hand on your heart: I LOVE YOU. YOU'VE GOT THIS, _____!
  (NAME)
- ∞ Affirmation: I (AM) _____
- ∞ I am grateful for (3+) _____
  _____
- ∞ I thank my body for _____
- ∞ HABIT TRACKER, Day ___ of 30

Wellbeing ACTIONS

- ☐ Today, I GET to _____ for me (prompts: JOY-FULL List p.15)
- ☐ Today, I GET to _____ my baby.
- ☐ Today, I GET to _____ for/with _____
  (e.g., spouse, kids, friends)

Nighttime REFLECTION

- ∞ WIN: I am *Celebrating* myself for _____
- ∞ CHALLENGE: It felt hard when _____
  - ♥ I choose to see this as an opportunity to _____
  - ♥ Say aloud: *I forgive, and I release this challenge with love.* *Inhale, Exhale*
- ∞ SUPPORT: I felt supported today by/when _____
  _____
- ∞ GRATITUDE: I am grateful for _____
  _____
- ∞ INTENTION: My intention for the morning is _____

Friday

Morning PEP TALK

- ∞ In the mirror, with one hand on your heart: I LOVE YOU. YOU'VE GOT THIS, _____!
  (NAME)
- ∞ Affirmation: I (AM) _____
- ∞ I am grateful for (3+) _____
  _____
- ∞ I thank my body for _____
- ∞ HABIT TRACKER, Day ___ of 30

Wellbeing ACTIONS

- ☐ Today, I GET to _____ for me (prompts: JOY-FULL List p.15)
- ☐ Today, I GET to _____ my baby.
- ☐ Today, I GET to _____ for/with _____
  (e.g., spouse, kids, friends)

Nighttime REFLECTION

- ∞ WIN: I am <u>Celebrating</u> myself for _____
- ∞ CHALLENGE: It felt hard when _____
  - ♥ I choose to see this as an opportunity to _____
  - ♥ Say aloud: *I forgive, and I release this challenge with love.*
    Inhale, Exhale
- ∞ SUPPORT: I felt supported today by/when _____
  _____
- ∞ GRATITUDE: I am grateful for _____
  _____
- ∞ INTENTION: My intention for the morning is _____

Saturday

Morning PEP TALK

- ∞ In the mirror, with one hand on your heart: I LOVE YOU. YOU'VE GOT THIS, _____ !
  (NAME)
- ∞ Affirmation: I (AM) _____
- ∞ I am grateful for (3+) _____
  _____
- ∞ I thank my body for _____
- ∞ HABIT TRACKER, Day ___ of 30

Wellbeing ACTIONS

- ☐ Today, I GET to _____ for me (prompts: JOY-FULL List p.15)
- ☐ Today, I GET to _____ my baby.
- ☐ Today, I GET to _____ for/with _____
  (e.g., spouse, kids, friends)

Nighttime REFLECTION

- ∞ WIN: I am <u>Celebrating</u> myself for _____
- ∞ CHALLENGE: It felt hard when _____
  - ♥ I choose to see this as an opportunity to _____
  - ♥ Say aloud: *I forgive, and I release this challenge with love. *Inhale, Exhale**
- ∞ SUPPORT: I felt supported today by/when _____
  _____
- ∞ GRATITUDE: I am grateful for _____
  _____
- ∞ INTENTION: My intention for the morning is _____

Sunday

Morning PEP TALK

- ∞ In the mirror, with one hand on your heart: I LOVE YOU. YOU'VE GOT THIS, _____!
  (NAME)
- ∞ Affirmation: I (AM) _____
- ∞ I am grateful for (3+) _____
  _____
- ∞ I thank my body for _____
- ∞ HABIT TRACKER, Day ___ of 30

Wellbeing ACTIONS

- ☐ Today, I GET to _____ for me (prompts: JOY-FULL List p.15)
- ☐ Today, I GET to _____ my baby.
- ☐ Today, I GET to _____ for/with _____
  (e.g., spouse, kids, friends)

Nighttime REFLECTION

- ∞ WIN: I am *Celebrating* myself for _____
- ∞ CHALLENGE: It felt hard when _____
  - ♥ I choose to see this as an opportunity to _____
  - ♥ Say aloud: *I forgive, and I release this challenge with love. *Inhale, Exhale**
- ∞ SUPPORT: I felt supported today by/when _____
  _____
- ∞ GRATITUDE: I am grateful for _____
  _____
- ∞ INTENTION: My intention for the morning is _____

Monthly Recap

- I am Celebrating _____!
    - ◊ In my head, I feel _____
    - ◊ In my heart, I feel _____
    - ◊ In my body, I feel _____
- My favourite activities this month were _____
  _____
    because _____
- My favourite affirmations this month were _____
  _____
    because _____
- It felt hard when _____
    From this, I learned _____
- I feel more joy and ease in my life when I _____
  _____
- I felt most supported this month when _____
- I am grateful for _____
- The boundary I set up at the beginning of the month helped me by
  _____
- I am celebrating my new habit this month!
    I am bringing this new habit with me into next month because (impact)
    _____
- Special milestones/memories (date and event):

MONTH:

Free write/Notes/Lessons/Draw

Reflections on the past 18 weeks

Let's Celebrate!

Cheers to you, Mama!

If you are reading this, *Congratulations*! What you have accomplished over these last four months in your postpartum journey is worthy of massive celebration. Whether you completed one day, every day, or somewhere in between, CELEBRATE – you have grown leaps and bounds and have come to know yourself more intimately as you've navigated this stage of your life.

If you feel you've benefited from this planner, we invite you to continue celebrating and tracking your journey with *The New Mama Celebration Planner*. It is a joy to share what we love! Who in your life do you want to thrive alongside with? Consider gifting one to that someone special. Our hope is that through gentle nudges to *Celebrate Yourself* EACH DAY and to grow from experiences that don't feel so good, all new mamas have the opportunity to *feel* and *be* supported in postpartum, and connected to their inner truth – together, we thrive.

Cheers to feeling more confidence and joy in your daily life. *Cheers* to showing up for yourself, your loved ones, and the world, every single day, however that looks.

Shine bright!

With Love and Gratitude,

Heather xo

Life is a celebration,
EVERY. SINGLE. DAY.

CPSIA information can be obtained
at www.ICGtesting.com
Printed in the USA
LVHW080458160822
726067LV00003B/17